MIDWIFERY

Record Book

MSc (Nursing) Ist Year

MIDWIFERY

Record Book

MSc (Nursing) Ist Year

(With Special Notes on Picture Representation of Midwifery, Investigations, Standard Values, Nursing Diagnosis, and Theories in Obstetrics and Gynecology)

R Lakshmi Devi MSc (Nursing)

Principal
Dhanwantari Nursing College
Bengaluru, Karnataka, India

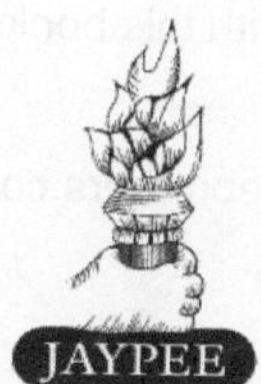

JAYPEE

JAYPEE BROTHERS MEDICAL PUBLISHERS

The Health Sciences Publisher

New Delhi | London

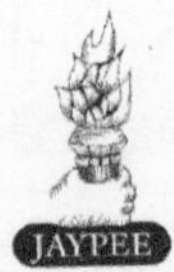

Jaypee Brothers Medical Publishers (P) Ltd.

Headquarters

EMCA House
23/23-B, Ansari Road, Daryaganj
New Delhi 110 002, India
Landline: +91-11-23272143,
+91-11-23272703+91-11-23282021,
+91-11-23245672
E-mail: jaypee@jaypeebrothers.com

Corporate Office

Jaypee Brothers Medical Publishers (P) Ltd.
4838/24, Ansari Road, Daryaganj
New Delhi 110 002, India
Phone: +91-11-43574357
Fax: +91-11-43574314
E-mail: jaypee@jaypeebrothers.com

Overseas Off ce

JP Medical Ltd.
83, Victoria Street, London
SW1H 0HW (UK)
Phone: +44-20 3170 8910
E-mail: info@jpmedpub.com

EU GPSR Authorised Representative

Logos Europe, 9 rue Nicolas Poussin
17000, La Rochelle, France
Phone: +33 (0) 6 67 93 73 78
E-mail: Contact@logoseurope.eu

Website: www.jaypeebrothers.com
Website: www.jaypeedigital.com

Inquiries for bulk sales may be solicited at: jaypee@jaypeebrothers.com

Midwifery Record Book: MSc (Nursing) Ist Year

First Edition: 2013
Reprint: **2025**
ISBN 978-93-5090-321-6

Printed in India

Dedicated to

If I had a flower for each time I thought of

my mother, I could walk in my garden forever,

and

All the mothers in the world.

PREFACE

Obstetrics and Gynecological Nursing are expanding areas as a result of the broadening scope of practice within the nursing profession and the recognized need for better preventive and restorative care in these areas.

The book is designed for MSc (Nursing) Ist Year students according to the revised syllabus (2009) formats for assessment, care plan and case study are included which deal with normal pregnancy.

A special notes on midwifery and gynecology with picture representation, standard table values, investigations, nursing diagnosis, and theories in obstetrics and gynecology are also included in the book.

I wish that the practical record book will be helpful for MSc (Nursing) Ist Year students to complete the practical requirements and develop a comprehensive skill in this field.

R Lakshmi Devi

ACKNOWLEDGMENTS

I owe a great deal of thanks to many who encouraged me with their time and efforts throughout the book.

My gratitude to my parents, my husband and my children for their support to finish this work and grateful thanks are extended to Mr Arif Ahmed (Chairman), Dhanwantari Nursing College, Bengaluru, Karnataka, India. My sincere thanks to my colleagues, students and friends who were with me during this work are Mr Muthuraja, Mrs Anjali, Ms Shanthi, Mrs Lakshmi, Mrs Muthu Kannu and Mr Nanda Kumar. I am also grateful to M/s Jaypee Brothers Medical Publishers (P) Ltd, New Delhi, India, who had given me an opportunity to pursue the book in the hands of students.

CONTENTS

Formats for Assessment 1

- Ist Year MSc Nursing Requirements Index 3-6
- Antenatal Assessment 8-27
- Intranatal Assessment 28-47
- Postnatal Assessment 48-67
- Conduct of Normal Delivery 68-267
- Perform Episiotomy and Suturing 268-277
- Insertion IUD 278-282

Antenatal Care Plan with Nursing Theory Application 283

- Antenatal Care Plan 285-368

Natal Care Plan with Nursing Theory Application 369

- Natal Care Plan 371-468

Postnatal Care Plan with Nursing Theory Application 469

- Postnatal Care Plan 471-523

Newborn Care Plan with Theory Application 525

- Newborn Care Plan 527-554

Gynecology Care Plan with Nursing Theory Application 555

- Gynecology Care Plan 557-572

Family Planning Care Plan with Nursing Theory Application 573

- Family Planning Care Plan 575-587

Antenatal Case Study 589-609

Natal Case Study 611-634

Postnatal Case Study 635-659

Newborn Case Study 661-680

Gynecology Case Study 681-702

- Clinical Specialty-I (Obstetric and Gynecological Nursing) 703-706

Special Notes 707-766

MIDWIFERY RECORD BOOK

MSc NURSING

Name of the College:____

Name of the Student:____

Register Number:____

Affix the Passport Size Photo

The practical work record is submitted towards the fulfillment of the requirement for the MSc degree in nursing

1ST YEAR MSc NURSING REQUIREMENTS INDEX

S. No.	Name of the Mother	Date	Signature of the Supervisor
ANTENATAL ASSESSMENT			
1.			
2.			
3.			
4.			
5.			
6.			
7.			
8.			
9.			
10.			
11.			
12.			
13.			
14.			
15.			
16.			
17.			
18.			
19.			
20.			
INTRANATAL ASSESSMENT			
1.			
2.			
3.			
4.			
5.			
6.			
7.			
8.			
9.			
10.			
11.			
12.			
13.			
14.			
15.			
16.			
17.			
18.			

19.			
20.			
POSTNATAL ASSESSMENT			
1.			
2.			
3.			
4.			
5.			
6.			
7.			
8.			
9.			
10.			
11.			
12.			
13.			
14.			
15.			
16.			
17.			
18.			
19.			
20.			
CONDUCT OF NORMAL DELIVERY			
1.			
2.			
3.			
4.			
5.			
6.			
7.			
8.			
9.			
10.			
11.			
12.			
13.			
14.			
15.			
16.			
17.			
18.			
19.			
20.			

PERFORM EPISIOTOMY AND SUTURING			
1.			
2.			
3.			
4.			
5.			
6.			
7.			
8.			
9.			
10.			
INSERTION OF IUD			
1.			
2.			
3.			
4.			
5.			
CARE PLAN WITH NURSING THEORY APPLICATION			
ANTENATAL			
1.			
2.			
3.			
4.			
5.			
NATAL			
1.			
2.			
3.			
4.			
5.			
POSTNATAL/GYNEC/FP			
1.			
2.			
3.			
4.			
5.			
NEWBORN			
1.			
2.			
CASE STUDY			
ANTENATAL			
1.			
NATAL			
1.			

I Year

POSTNATAL			
1.			
NEWBORN			
1.			
GYNECOLOGY			
1.			

---------------------- Signature of the Student

--------------------- Signature of the HOD

--------------------- Signature of the Principal

Signature of the Examiner:

--------------------- Internal

--------------------- External

ANTENATAL ASSESSMENT

						General Examination								
S. No.	Date of Assessment	Name and Age	Gravida	PARA	LMP/EDD	Height	Weight	Heart	Lungs	BP	Breast Examination	Abdomen	Perineum	Legs and Feet

Obstetrical Examination				Symptoms					
Gestational Age	Height of Fundus	Abdominal Girth	Presentation Position	FHR	Pain	Appetite	Heart Burn	Micturition	Nursing Care

I Year

ANTENATAL ASSESSMENT

						General Examination								
S. No.	Date of Assessment	Name and Age	Gravida	PARA	LMP/EDD	Height	Weight	Heart	Lungs	BP	Breast Examination	Abdomen	Perineum	Legs and Feet

Obstetrical Examination				Symptoms					
Gestational Age	Height of Fundus	Abdominal Girth	Presentation Position	FHR	Pain	Appetite	Heart Burn	Micturition	Nursing Care

I Year

ANTENATAL ASSESSMENT

S. No.	Date of Assessment	Name and Age	Gravida	PARA	LMP/EDD	General Examination									
						Height	Weight	Heart	Lungs	BP	Breast Examination	Abdomen	Perineum	Legs and Feet

Obstetrical Examination				Symptoms					
Gestational Age	Height of Fundus	Abdominal Girth	Presentation Position	FHR	Pain	Appetite	Heart Burn	Micturition	Nursing Care

ANTENATAL ASSESSMENT

						General Examination								
S. No.	Date of Assessment	Name and Age	Gravida	PARA	LMP/EDD	Height	Weight	Heart	Lungs	BP	Breast Examination	Abdomen	Perineum	Legs and Feet

Obstetrical Examination				Symptoms					
Gestational Age	Height of Fundus	Abdominal Girth	Presentation Position	FHR	Pain	Appetite	Heart Burn	Micturition	Nursing Care

I Year

ANTENATAL ASSESSMENT

						General Examination								
S. No.	Date of Assessment	Name and Age	Gravida	PARA	LMP/EDD	Height	Weight	Heart	Lungs	BP	Breast Examination	Abdomen	Perineum	Legs and Feet

Obstetrical Examination				Symptoms					
Gestational Age	Height of Fundus	Abdominal Girth	Presentation Position	FHR	Pain	Appetite	Heart Burn	Micturition	Nursing Care

I Year

ANTENATAL ASSESSMENT

						General Examination								
S. No.	Date of Assessment	Name and Age	Gravida	PARA	LMP/EDD	Height	Weight	Heart	Lungs	BP	Breast Examination	Abdomen	Perineum	Legs and Feet

Obstetrical Examination				Symptoms					
Gestational Age	Height of Fundus	Abdominal Girth	Presentation Position	FHR	Pain	Appetite	Heart Burn	Micturition	Nursing Care

ANTENATAL ASSESSMENT

						General Examination								
S. No.	Date of Assessment	Name and Age	Gravida	PARA	LMP/EDD	Height	Weight	Heart	Lungs	BP	Breast Examination	Abdomen	Perineum	Legs and Feet

Obstetrical Examination				Symptoms					
Gestational Age	Height of Fundus	Abdominal Girth	Presentation Position	FHR	Pain	Appetite	Heart Burn	Micturition	Nursing Care

I Year

ANTENATAL ASSESSMENT

						General Examination								
S. No.	Date of Assessment	Name and Age	Gravida	PARA	LMP/EDD	Height	Weight	Heart	Lungs	BP	Breast Examination	Abdomen	Perineum	Legs and Feet

Obstetrical Examination				Symptoms					
Gestational Age	Height of Fundus	Abdominal Girth	Presentation Position	FHR	Pain	Appetite	Heart Burn	Micturition	Nursing Care

ANTENATAL ASSESSMENT

						General Examination								
S. No.	Date of Assessment	Name and Age	Gravida	PARA	LMP/EDD	Height	Weight	Heart	Lungs	BP	Breast Examination	Abdomen	Perineum	Legs and Feet

Obstetrical Examination				Symptoms					
Gestational Age	Height of Fundus	Abdominal Girth	Presentation Position	FHR	Pain	Appetite	Heart Burn	Micturition	Nursing Care

ANTENATAL ASSESSMENT

						General Examination								
S. No.	Date of Assessment	Name and Age	Gravida	PARA	LMP/EDD	Height	Weight	Heart	Lungs	BP	Breast Examination	Abdomen	Perineum	Legs and Feet

Obstetrical Examination				Symptoms					
Gestational Age	Height of Fundus	Abdominal Girth	Presentation Position	FHR	Pain	Appetite	Heart Burn	Micturition	Nursing Care

I Year

INTRANATAL ASSESSMENT

S. No.	Date of Assessment	Name and Age	Gravida	PARA	LMP/PEDD	Admission Date	Time	Period of Gestation	Contraction commenced at	Special Observation
										Temperature Pulse Blood Pressure FHR Contractions Cervical Dilatation Position Effacement Drugs Intake Output Nurses Role

Time					Delivery Notes	Delivery of Placenta	Nursing Care/ Discharge Summary
					Membrane Ruptured at	Normal/Manually Removed at	
					Spontaneously/Artificially	Examination of Placenta	
					Reason	Weight of Placenta	
					Expulsive Contraction	Cord insertion/Length	
					Baby Born at	Maternal Surface	
					Condition when at Born	Fetal Surface	
					Alive/Asphyxiated/Stillbirth/Macerated	Blood Loss	
					Sex of the Baby	Condition of Perineum	
					Care of the Baby	Episiotomy	
					Apgar Score	Intact/Tear	
					Weight	Repaires	
					Height	**Condition/Care of Mother**	
					General Observation	Pulse	
					Cord ligation	BP	
					Cord Care	Fundal Height	
					Baby Bath	Uterus Soft/Hard	
					Initiation of Breast Feeding	Vaginal Bleeding Normal/Abnormal	

INTRANATAL ASSESSMENT

S. No.	Date of Assessment	Name and Age	Gravida	PARA	LMP/PEDD	Admission Date	Time	Period of Gestation	Contraction commenced at	Special Observation
										Temperature Pulse Blood Pressure FHR Contractions Cervical Dilatation Position Effacement Drugs Intake Output Nurses Role

Time					Delivery Notes	Delivery of Placenta	Nursing Care/ Discharge Summary
					Membrane Ruptured at	Normal/Manually Removed at	
					Spontaneously/Artificially	Examination of Placenta	
					Reason	Weight of Placenta	
					Expulsive Contraction	Cord insertion/Length	
					Baby Born at	Maternal Surface	
					Condition when at Born	Fetal Surface	
					Alive/Asphyxiated/Stillbirth/Macerated	Blood Loss	
					Sex of the Baby	Condition of Perineum	
					Care of the Baby	Episiotomy	
					Apgar Score	Intact/Tear	
					Weight	Repaires	
					Height	**Condition/Care of Mother**	
					General Observation	Pulse	
					Cord ligation	BP	
					Cord Care	Fundal Height	
					Baby Bath	Uterus Soft/Hard	
					Initiation of Breast Feeding	Vaginal Bleeding Normal/Abnormal	

INTRANATAL ASSESSMENT

S. No.	Date of Assessment	Name and Age	Gravida	PARA	LMP/PEDD	Admission Date	Time	Period of Gestation	Contraction commenced at	Special Observation
										Temperature Pulse Blood Pressure FHR Contractions Cervical Dilatation Position Effacement Drugs Intake Output Nurses Role

Time					Delivery Notes	Delivery of Placenta	Nursing Care/ Discharge Summary
					Membrane Ruptured at	Normal/Manually Removed at	
					Spontaneously/Artificially	Examination of Placenta	
					Reason	Weight of Placenta	
					Expulsive Contraction	Cord insertion/Length	
					Baby Born at	Maternal Surface	
					Condition when at Born	Fetal Surface	
					Alive/Asphyxiated/Stillbirth/Macerated	Blood Loss	
					Sex of the Baby	Condition of Perineum	
					Care of the Baby	Episiotomy	
					Apgar Score	Intact/Tear	
					Weight	Repaires	
					Height	**Condition/Care of Mother**	
					General Observation	Pulse	
					Cord ligation	BP	
					Cord Care	Fundal Height	
					Baby Bath	Uterus Soft/Hard	
					Initiation of Breast Feeding	Vaginal Bleeding Normal/Abnormal	

INTRANATAL ASSESSMENT

S. No.	Date of Assessment	Name and Age	Gravida	PARA	LMP/PEDD	Admission Date	Time	Period of Gestation	Contraction commenced at	Special Observation
										Temperature Pulse Blood Pressure FHR Contractions Cervical Dilatation Position Effacement Drugs Intake Output Nurses Role

Time					Delivery Notes	Delivery of Placenta	Nursing Care/ Discharge Summary
					Membrane Ruptured at Spontaneously/Artificially Reason Expulsive Contraction Baby Born at Condition when at Born Alive/Asphyxiated/Stillbirth/Macerated Sex of the Baby **Care of the Baby** Apgar Score Weight Height General Observation Cord ligation Cord Care Baby Bath Initiation of Breast Feeding	Normal/Manually Removed at Examination of Placenta Weight of Placenta Cord insertion/Length Maternal Surface Fetal Surface Blood Loss Condition of Perineum Episiotomy Intact/Tear Repaires **Condition/Care of Mother** Pulse BP Fundal Height Uterus Soft/Hard Vaginal Bleeding Normal/Abnormal	

INTRANATAL ASSESSMENT

S. No.	Date of Assessment	Name and Age	Gravida	PARA	LMP/PEDD	Admission Date	Time	Period of Gestation	Contraction commenced at	Special Observation
										Temperature Pulse Blood Pressure FHR Contractions Cervical Dilatation Position Effacement Drugs Intake Output Nurses Role

Time					Delivery Notes	Delivery of Placenta	Nursing Care/ Discharge Summary
					Membrane Ruptured at	Normal/Manually Removed at	
					Spontaneously/Artificially	Examination of Placenta	
					Reason	Weight of Placenta	
					Expulsive Contraction	Cord insertion/Length	
					Baby Born at	Maternal Surface	
					Condition when at Born	Fetal Surface	
					Alive/Asphyxiated/Stillbirth/Macerated	Blood Loss	
					Sex of the Baby	Condition of Perineum	
					Care of the Baby	Episiotomy	
					Apgar Score	Intact/Tear	
					Weight	Repaires	
					Height	**Condition/Care of Mother**	
					General Observation	Pulse	
					Cord ligation	BP	
					Cord Care	Fundal Height	
					Baby Bath	Uterus Soft/Hard	
					Initiation of Breast Feeding	Vaginal Bleeding Normal/Abnormal	

INTRANATAL ASSESSMENT

S. No.	Date of Assessment	Name and Age	Gravida	PARA	LMP/PEDD	Admission Date	Time	Period of Gestation	Contraction commenced at	Special Observation
										Temperature Pulse Blood Pressure FHR Contractions Cervical Dilatation Position Effacement Drugs Intake Output Nurses Role

Time					Delivery Notes	Delivery of Placenta	Nursing Care/ Discharge Summary
					Membrane Ruptured at	Normal/Manually Removed at	
					Spontaneously/Artificially	Examination of Placenta	
					Reason	Weight of Placenta	
					Expulsive Contraction	Cord insertion/Length	
					Baby Born at	Maternal Surface	
					Condition when at Born	Fetal Surface	
					Alive/Asphyxiated/Stillbirth/Macerated	Blood Loss	
					Sex of the Baby	Condition of Perineum	
					Care of the Baby	Episiotomy	
					Apgar Score	Intact/Tear	
					Weight	Repaires	
					Height	**Condition/Care of Mother**	
					General Observation	Pulse	
					Cord ligation	BP	
					Cord Care	Fundal Height	
					Baby Bath	Uterus Soft/Hard	
					Initiation of Breast Feeding	Vaginal Bleeding Normal/Abnormal	

INTRANATAL ASSESSMENT

S. No.	Date of Assessment	Name and Age	Gravida	PARA	LMP/PEDD	Admission Date	Time	Period of Gestation	Contraction commenced at	Special Observation
										Temperature Pulse Blood Pressure FHR Contractions Cervical Dilatation Position Effacement Drugs Intake Output Nurses Role

Time					Delivery Notes	Delivery of Placenta	Nursing Care/ Discharge Summary
					Membrane Ruptured at	Normal/Manually Removed at	
					Spontaneously/Artificially	Examination of Placenta	
					Reason	Weight of Placenta	
					Expulsive Contraction	Cord insertion/Length	
					Baby Born at	Maternal Surface	
					Condition when at Born	Fetal Surface	
					Alive/Asphyxiated/Stillbirth/Macerated	Blood Loss	
					Sex of the Baby	Condition of Perineum	
					Care of the Baby	Episiotomy	
					Apgar Score	Intact/Tear	
					Weight	Repaires	
					Height	**Condition/Care of Mother**	
					General Observation	Pulse	
					Cord ligation	BP	
					Cord Care	Fundal Height	
					Baby Bath	Uterus Soft/Hard	
					Initiation of Breast Feeding	Vaginal Bleeding Normal/Abnormal	

INTRANATAL ASSESSMENT

S. No.	Date of Assessment	Name and Age	Gravida	PARA	LMP/PEDD	Admission Date	Time	Period of Gestation	Contraction commenced at	Special Observation
										Temperature Pulse Blood Pressure FHR Contractions Cervical Dilatation Position Effacement Drugs Intake Output Nurses Role

Time					Delivery Notes	Delivery of Placenta	Nursing Care/ Discharge Summary
					Membrane Ruptured at	Normal/Manually Removed at	
					Spontaneously/Artificially	Examination of Placenta	
					Reason	Weight of Placenta	
					Expulsive Contraction	Cord insertion/Length	
					Baby Born at	Maternal Surface	
					Condition when at Born	Fetal Surface	
					Alive/Asphyxiated/Stillbirth/Macerated	Blood Loss	
					Sex of the Baby	Condition of Perineum	
					Care of the Baby	Episiotomy	
					Apgar Score	Intact/Tear	
					Weight	Repaires	
					Height	**Condition/Care of Mother**	
					General Observation	Pulse	
					Cord ligation	BP	
					Cord Care	Fundal Height	
					Baby Bath	Uterus Soft/Hard	
					Initiation of Breast Feeding	Vaginal Bleeding Normal/Abnormal	

INTRANATAL ASSESSMENT

S. No.	Date of Assessment	Name and Age	Gravida	PARA	LMP/PEDD	Admission Date	Time	Period of Gestation	Contraction commenced at	Special Observation
										Temperature Pulse Blood Pressure FHR Contractions Cervical Dilatation Position Effacement Drugs Intake Output Nurses Role

Time					Delivery Notes	Delivery of Placenta	Nursing Care/ Discharge Summary
					Membrane Ruptured at Spontaneously/Artificially Reason Expulsive Contraction Baby Born at Condition when at Born Alive/Asphyxiated/Stillbirth/Macerated Sex of the Baby **Care of the Baby** Apgar Score Weight Height General Observation Cord ligation Cord Care Baby Bath Initiation of Breast Feeding	Normal/Manually Removed at Examination of Placenta Weight of Placenta Cord insertion/Length Maternal Surface Fetal Surface Blood Loss Condition of Perineum Episiotomy Intact/Tear Repaires **Condition/Care of Mother** Pulse BP Fundal Height Uterus Soft/Hard Vaginal Bleeding Normal/Abnormal	

I Year

INTRANATAL ASSESSMENT

S. No.	Date of Assessment	Name and Age	Gravida	PARA	LMP/PEDD	Admission Date	Time	Period of Gestation	Contraction commenced at	Special Observation
										Temperature Pulse Blood Pressure FHR Contractions Cervical Dilatation Position Effacement Drugs Intake Output Nurses Role

Time					Delivery Notes	Delivery of Placenta	Nursing Care/ Discharge Summary
					Membrane Ruptured at	Normal/Manually Removed at	
					Spontaneously/Artificially	Examination of Placenta	
					Reason	Weight of Placenta	
					Expulsive Contraction	Cord insertion/Length	
					Baby Born at	Maternal Surface	
					Condition when at Born	Fetal Surface	
					Alive/Asphyxiated/Stillbirth/Macerated	Blood Loss	
					Sex of the Baby	Condition of Perineum	
					Care of the Baby	Episiotomy	
					Apgar Score	Intact/Tear	
					Weight	Repaires	
					Height	**Condition/Care of Mother**	
					General Observation	Pulse	
					Cord ligation	BP	
					Cord Care	Fundal Height	
					Baby Bath	Uterus Soft/Hard	
					Initiation of Breast Feeding	Vaginal Bleeding Normal/Abnormal	

POSTNATAL ASSESSMENT

S. No.	Date of Assessment	Age	Gravida	PARA	Date of Delivery	Delivery Notes	Delivery of Placenta	Clinical Chart of Puerperium
						Membrane Ruptured at Spontaneously/Artificially Reason Expulsive Contraction Baby Born at Condition when at Born Alive/Asphyxiated/Stillbirth/Macerated Sex of the Baby *Care of the Baby* Apgar Score Weight Height General Observation Cord Ligation Cord Care Baby Bath Initiation of Breast Feeding	Normal/Manually Removed at Examination of Placenta Weight of Placenta Cord insertion/Length Maternal Surface Fetal Surface Blood Loss Condition of Perineum Episiotomy Intact/Tear Reo/Paired *Condition/Care of Mother* Pulse BP Fundal Height Uterus: Soft/Hard Vaginal Bleeding: Normal/Abnormal	Temperature Pulse Respiration BP Lochia Urine Motion

Date			Clinical Chart of Baby	Date			Nursing Care/Discharge Summary
			Temperature Heart Rate Respiration Urine Stool Vomit Jaundice Weight Umbilical Core				

I Year

POSTNATAL ASSESSMENT

S. No.	Date of Assessment	Age	Gravida	PARA	Date of Delivery	Delivery Notes	Delivery of Placenta	Clinical Chart of Puerperium
						Membrane Ruptured at Spontaneously/Artificially Reason Expulsive Contraction Baby Born at Condition when at Born Alive/Asphyxiated/Stillbirth/Macerated Sex of the Baby ***Care of the Baby*** Apgar Score Weight Height General Observation Cord Ligation Cord Care Baby Bath Initiation of Breast Feeding	Normal/Manually Removed at Examination of Placenta Weight of Placenta Cord insertion/Length Maternal Surface Fetal Surface Blood Loss Condition of Perineum Episiotomy Intact/Tear Reo/Paired ***Condition/Care of Mother*** Pulse BP Fundal Height Uterus: Soft/Hard Vaginal Bleeding: Normal/Abnormal	Temperature Pulse Respiration BP Lochia Urine Motion

Date			Clinical Chart of Baby	Date			Nursing Care/Discharge Summary
			Temperature				
			Heart Rate				
			Respiration				
			Urine				
			Stool				
			Vomit				
			Jaundice				
			Weight				
			Umbilical Core				

I Year

POSTNATAL ASSESSMENT

S. No.	Date of Assessment	Age	Gravida	PARA	Date of Delivery	Delivery Notes	Delivery of Placenta	Clinical Chart of Puerperium
						Membrane Ruptured at Spontaneously/Artificially Reason Expulsive Contraction Baby Born at Condition when at Born Alive/Asphyxiated/Stillbirth/Macerated Sex of the Baby ***Care of the Baby*** Apgar Score Weight Height General Observation Cord Ligation Cord Care Baby Bath Initiation of Breast Feeding	Normal/Manually Removed at Examination of Placenta Weight of Placenta Cord insertion/Length Maternal Surface Fetal Surface Blood Loss Condition of Perineum Episiotomy Intact/Tear Reo/Paired ***Condition/Care of Mother*** Pulse BP Fundal Height Uterus: Soft/Hard Vaginal Bleeding: Normal/Abnormal	Temperature Pulse Respiration BP Lochia Urine Motion

Date			Clinical Chart of Baby	Date			Nursing Care/Discharge Summary
			Temperature				
			Heart Rate				
			Respiration				
			Urine				
			Stool				
			Vomit				
			Jaundice				
			Weight				
			Umbilical Core				

POSTNATAL ASSESSMENT

S. No.	Date of Assessment	Age	Gravida	PARA	Date of Delivery	Delivery Notes	Delivery of Placenta	Clinical Chart of Puerperium
						Membrane Ruptured at Spontaneously/Artificially Reason Expulsive Contraction Baby Born at Condition when at Born Alive/Asphyxiated/Stillbirth/Macerated Sex of the Baby ***Care of the Baby*** Apgar Score Weight Height General Observation Cord Ligation Cord Care Baby Bath Initiation of Breast Feeding	Normal/Manually Removed at Examination of Placenta Weight of Placenta Cord insertion/Length Maternal Surface Fetal Surface Blood Loss Condition of Perineum Episiotomy Intact/Tear Reo/Paired ***Condition/Care of Mother*** Pulse BP Fundal Height Uterus: Soft/Hard Vaginal Bleeding: Normal/Abnormal	Temperature Pulse Respiration BP Lochia Urine Motion

Date			Clinical Chart of Baby	Date			Nursing Care/Discharge Summary
			Temperature Heart Rate Respiration Urine Stool Vomit Jaundice Weight Umbilical Core				

I Year

POSTNATAL ASSESSMENT

S. No.	Date of Assessment	Age	Gravida	PARA	Date of Delivery	Delivery Notes	Delivery of Placenta	Clinical Chart of Puerperium
						Membrane Ruptured at Spontaneously/Artificially Reason Expulsive Contraction Baby Born at Condition when at Born Alive/Asphyxiated/Stillbirth/Macerated Sex of the Baby *Care of the Baby* Apgar Score Weight Height General Observation Cord Ligation Cord Care Baby Bath Initiation of Breast Feeding	Normal/Manually Removed at Examination of Placenta Weight of Placenta Cord insertion/Length Maternal Surface Fetal Surface Blood Loss Condition of Perineum Episiotomy Intact/Tear Reo/Paired *Condition/Care of Mother* Pulse BP Fundal Height Uterus: Soft/Hard Vaginal Bleeding: Normal/Abnormal	Temperature Pulse Respiration BP Lochia Urine Motion

Date			Clinical Chart of Baby	Date			Nursing Care/Discharge Summary
			Temperature Heart Rate Respiration Urine Stool Vomit Jaundice Weight Umbilical Core				

POSTNATAL ASSESSMENT

S. No.	Date of Assessment	Age	Gravida	PARA	Date of Delivery	Delivery Notes	Delivery of Placenta	Clinical Chart of Puerperium
						Membrane Ruptured at Spontaneously/Artificially Reason Expulsive Contraction Baby Born at Condition when at Born Alive/Asphyxiated/Stillbirth/Macerated Sex of the Baby ***Care of the Baby*** Apgar Score Weight Height General Observation Cord Ligation Cord Care Baby Bath Initiation of Breast Feeding	Normal/Manually Removed at Examination of Placenta Weight of Placenta Cord insertion/Length Maternal Surface Fetal Surface Blood Loss Condition of Perineum Episiotomy Intact/Tear Reo/Paired ***Condition/Care of Mother*** Pulse BP Fundal Height Uterus: Soft/Hard Vaginal Bleeding: Normal/Abnormal	Temperature Pulse Respiration BP Lochia Urine Motion

Date			Clinical Chart of Baby	Date			Nursing Care/Discharge Summary
			Temperature Heart Rate Respiration Urine Stool Vomit Jaundice Weight Umbilical Core				

I Year

POSTNATAL ASSESSMENT

S. No.	Date of Assessment	Age	Gravida	PARA	Date of Delivery	Delivery Notes	Delivery of Placenta	Clinical Chart of Puerperium
						Membrane Ruptured at Spontaneously/Artificially Reason Expulsive Contraction Baby Born at Condition when at Born Alive/Asphyxiated/Stillbirth/Macerated Sex of the Baby ***Care of the Baby*** Apgar Score Weight Height General Observation Cord Ligation Cord Care Baby Bath Initiation of Breast Feeding	Normal/Manually Removed at Examination of Placenta Weight of Placenta Cord insertion/Length Maternal Surface Fetal Surface Blood Loss Condition of Perineum Episiotomy Intact/Tear Reo/Paired ***Condition/Care of Mother*** Pulse BP Fundal Height Uterus: Soft/Hard Vaginal Bleeding: Normal/Abnormal	Temperature Pulse Respiration BP Lochia Urine Motion

Date			Clinical Chart of Baby	Date			Nursing Care/Discharge Summary
			Temperature Heart Rate Respiration Urine Stool Vomit Jaundice Weight Umbilical Core				

I Year

POSTNATAL ASSESSMENT

S. No.	Date of Assessment	Age	Gravida	PARA	Date of Delivery	Delivery Notes	Delivery of Placenta	Clinical Chart of Puerperium
						Membrane Ruptured at Spontaneously/Artificially Reason Expulsive Contraction Baby Born at Condition when at Born Alive/Asphyxiated/Stillbirth/Macerated Sex of the Baby ***Care of the Baby*** Apgar Score Weight Height General Observation Cord Ligation Cord Care Baby Bath Initiation of Breast Feeding	Normal/Manually Removed at Examination of Placenta Weight of Placenta Cord insertion/Length Maternal Surface Fetal Surface Blood Loss Condition of Perineum Episiotomy Intact/Tear Reo/Paired ***Condition/Care of Mother*** Pulse BP Fundal Height Uterus: Soft/Hard Vaginal Bleeding: Normal/Abnormal	Temperature Pulse Respiration BP Lochia Urine Motion

Date			Clinical Chart of Baby	Date			Nursing Care/Discharge Summary
			Temperature Heart Rate Respiration Urine Stool Vomit Jaundice Weight Umbilical Core				

I Year

POSTNATAL ASSESSMENT

S. No.	Date of Assessment	Age	Gravida	PARA	Date of Delivery	Delivery Notes	Delivery of Placenta	Clinical Chart of Puerperium
						Membrane Ruptured at Spontaneously/Artificially Reason Expulsive Contraction Baby Born at Condition when at Born Alive/Asphyxiated/Stillbirth/Macerated Sex of the Baby ***Care of the Baby*** Apgar Score Weight Height General Observation Cord Ligation Cord Care Baby Bath Initiation of Breast Feeding	Normal/Manually Removed at Examination of Placenta Weight of Placenta Cord insertion/Length Maternal Surface Fetal Surface Blood Loss Condition of Perineum Episiotomy Intact/Tear Reo/Paired ***Condition/Care of Mother*** Pulse BP Fundal Height Uterus: Soft/Hard Vaginal Bleeding: Normal/Abnormal	Temperature Pulse Respiration BP Lochia Urine Motion

Date			Clinical Chart of Baby	Date			Nursing Care/Discharge Summary
			Temperature Heart Rate Respiration Urine Stool Vomit Jaundice Weight Umbilical Core				

POSTNATAL ASSESSMENT

S. No.	Date of Assessment	Age	Gravida	PARA	Date of Delivery	Delivery Notes	Delivery of Placenta	Clinical Chart of Puerperium
						Membrane Ruptured at Spontaneously/Artificially Reason Expulsive Contraction Baby Born at Condition when at Born Alive/Asphyxiated/Stillbirth/Macerated Sex of the Baby *Care of the Baby* Apgar Score Weight Height General Observation Cord Ligation Cord Care Baby Bath Initiation of Breast Feeding	Normal/Manually Removed at Examination of Placenta Weight of Placenta Cord insertion/Length Maternal Surface Fetal Surface Blood Loss Condition of Perineum Episiotomy Intact/Tear Reo/Paired *Condition/Care of Mother* Pulse BP Fundal Height Uterus: Soft/Hard Vaginal Bleeding: Normal/Abnormal	Temperature Pulse Respiration BP Lochia Urine Motion

Date			Clinical Chart of Baby	Date			Nursing Care/Discharge Summary
			Temperature Heart Rate Respiration Urine Stool Vomit Jaundice Weight Umbilical Core				

CONDUCT OF NORMAL DELIVERY

Name:

Age:

Hospital no:

Date of admission:

Date of delivery:

Prenatal record

Gravida:

PARA:

LMP:

EDD:

ANTENATAL ATTENDANCE

Date	Weight	Urine		BP mm of Hg	Fundal Height in cm	Gestational Age	FHR/Minute
		Alb.	Sugar				

INVESTIGATIONS /EXAMINATIONS

Blood group:

Hb:

Breasts:

Nipples:

General conditions:

OBSTETRICAL HISTORY

S. No.	Date	Abortion	Preterm	Fullterm	Type of Delivery	Sex	Alive/Stillbirth

ADMISSION TO LABOR ROOM

Admission on------------------------------at--------------------------am/pm.

Period of gestation:

Contraction commenced on--------------------at--------------am/pm.

Height of fundus:

Presentation:

Position:

Head: Engaged /not engaged

Nature of contraction:

FHR:

Bladder:

Bowel:

Vaginal examination

Effacement:

Cervix dilatation:

Station:

Membranes: Intact/ruptured on

Liquor:

DELIVERY NOTES

Membranes ruptured at -----------am/pm, on-------------------------------

Spontaneously/artificially

Reason:

Expulsive contraction commenced at --------am/pm, on------------baby.

Born at---------am/pm, on ----------------------

Sex of the baby:

Apgar Score:

Condition of baby at birth

Active/limp/asphyxiated

Alive/stillborn/macerated

Cause:

TREATMENT AT BIRTH

PLACENTA /MEMBRANES

Delivered at------------am/pm, on -------------------------

Spontaneously/helped/manually removed

Type of placenta; healthy/infarcts

Maternal side: Complete/incomplete

Fetal side:

Weight:

Cord insertion:

Cord length:

BLOOD LOSS

Before delivery of placenta ----------------

During delivery of placenta ----------------

After delivery of placenta ----------------

Total ----------------

CONDITION OF PERINEUM

Intact/episiotomy

Torn/degree

Repaired with

DRUGS GIVEN DURING DELIVERY

DRUGS GIVEN AFTER DELIVERY

LABOR SUMMARY

Type of labor:

Mode of delivery:

Length of labor

I stage of labor --------------hours ------------minutes

II stage of labor --------------hours ------------minutes

III stage of labor --------------hours ------------minutes

Total --------------hours ------------minutes

CONDITION OF THE MOTHER AFTER DELIVERY

Temperature:

Pulse:

Blood pressure:

Fundal height :

Uterus: Hard/soft

Vaginal Bleeding: Normal/abnormal

CLINICAL CHART OF PUERPERIUM

Date														
Temperature	M	E	M	E	M	E	M	E	M	E	M	E	M	E
Pulse														
Respiration														
Fundal Height														
Lochia														
Urine														
Motion														

CONDITION OF MOTHER /BABY ON DISCHARGE

Date			
Mother		Baby	
General condition		General condition	
Uterus		Weight	
Lochia		Length	
Episiotomy		Head circumference	
Breast		Chest circumference	
		Feeds	
		Urine/Stool	
		Date of cord separation	

INSTRUCTION ON DISCHARGE

CONDUCT OF NORMAL DELIVERY

Name:

Age:

Hospital no:

Date of admission:

Date of delivery:

Prenatal record

Gravida:

PARA:

LMP:

EDD:

ANTENATAL ATTENDANCE

Date	Weight	Urine		BP	Fundal Height	Gestational Age	FHR
		Alb.	Sugar				

INVESTIGATIONS /EXAMINATIONS

Blood group:

Hb:

Breasts:

Nipples:

General conditions:

OBSTETRICAL HISTORY

S. No.	Date	Abortion	Preterm	Fullterm	Type of Delivery	Sex	Alive/Stillbirth

ADMISSION TO LABOR ROOM

Admission on-----------------------------at-------------------------am/pm.

Period of gestation:

Contraction commenced on--------------------at--------------am/pm.

Height of fundus:

Presentation:

Position:

Head: Engaged /not engaged

Nature of contraction:

FHR:

Bladder:

Bowel:

Vaginal examination

Effacement:

Cervix dilatation:

Station:

Membranes: Intact/ruptured on

Liquor:

PARTOGRAM

I Year

DELIVERY NOTES

Membranes ruptured at ------------am/pm, on--------------------------------

Spontaneously/artificially

Reason:

Expulsive contraction commenced at --------am/pm, on------------baby.

Born at---------am/pm, on ----------------------

Sex of the baby:

Apgar Score:

Condition of baby at birth

Active/limp/asphyxiated

Alive/stillborn/macerated

Cause:

TREATMENT AT BIRTH

PLACENTA /MEMBRANES

Delivered at-----------am/pm, on ------------------------

Spontaneously /helped/manually removed

Type of placenta; healthy/infarcts

Maternal side: Complete/incomplete

Fetal side:

Weight:

Cord insertion:

Cord length:

BLOOD LOSS

Before delivery of placenta ---------------

During delivery of placenta ---------------

After delivery of placenta ---------------

Total ---------------

CONDITION OF PERINEUM

Intact/episiotomy

Torn/degree

Repaired with

DRUGS GIVEN DURING DELIVERY

DRUGS GIVEN AFTER DELIVERY

LABOR SUMMARY

Type of labor:

Mode of delivery :

Length of labor

I stage of labor --------------hours ------------minutes

II stage of labor --------------hours ------------minutes

III stage of labor --------------hours ------------minutes

Total --------------hours ------------minutes

CONDITION OF THE MOTHER AFTER DELIVERY

Temperature:

Pulse:

Blood pressure:

Fundal height :

Uterus:Hard/soft

Vaginal bleeding: Normal/abnormal

CLINICAL CHART OF PUERPERIUM

Date														
Temperature	M	E	M	E	M	E	M	E	M	E	M	E	M	E
Pulse														
Respiration														
Fundal Height														
Lochia														
Urine														
Motion														

CONDITION OF MOTHER /BABY ON DISCHARGE

Date			
Mother		Baby	
General condition		General condition	
Uterus		Weight	
Lochia		Length	
Episiotomy		Head circumference	
Breast		Chest circumference	
		Feeds	
		Urine/stool	
		Date of cord separation	

I Year

INSTRUCTION ON DISCHARGE

CONDUCT OF NORMAL DELIVERY

Name:

Age:

Hospital no:

Date of admission:

Date of delivery:

Prenatal record

Gravida:

PARA:

LMP:

EDD:

ANTENATAL ATTENDANCE

Date	Weight	Urine		BP	Fundal Height	Gestational Age	FHR
		Alb.	Sugar				

INVESTIGATIONS /EXAMINATIONS

Blood group:

Hb:

Breasts:

Nipples:

General conditions:

OBSTETRICAL HISTORY

S. No.	Date	Abortion	Preterm	Fullterm	Type of Delivery	Sex	Alive/Stillbirth

ADMISSION TO LABOR ROOM

Admission on-----------------------------at-------------------------am/pm.

Period of gestation:

Contraction commenced on-------------------at--------------am/pm.

Height of fundus:

Presentation:

Position:

Head: Engaged /not engaged

Nature of contraction:

FHR:

Bladder:

Bowel:

Vaginal examination

Effacement:

Cervix dilatation:

Station:

Membranes: Intact/ruptured on

Liquor:

DELIVERY NOTES

Membranes ruptured at ------------am/pm, on--------------------------------

Spontaneously/artificially

Reason:

Expulsive contraction commenced at --------am/pm, on-------------baby.

Born at----------am/pm, on ----------------------

Sex of the baby:

Apgar Score:

Condition of baby at birth

Active/limp/asphyxiated

Alive/stillborn/macerated

Cause:

TREATMENT AT BIRTH

PLACENTA /MEMBRANES

Delivered at-----------am/pm, on ------------------------

Spontaneously /helped/manually removed

Type of placenta; healthy/infarcts

Maternal side: Complete/Incomplete

Fetal side:

Weight:

Cord insertion:

Cord length:

BLOOD LOSS

Before delivery of placenta ----------------

During delivery of placenta ----------------

After delivery of placenta ----------------

Total ----------------

CONDITION OF PERINEUM

Intact/episiotomy

Torn/degree

Repaired with

DRUGS GIVEN DURING DELIVERY

DRUGS GIVEN AFTER DELIVERY

LABOR SUMMARY

Type of labor:

Mode of delivery:

Length of labor

I stage of labor ---------------hours ------------minutes

II stage of labor ---------------hours ------------minutes

III stage of labor ---------------hours ------------minutes

Total ---------------hours ------------minutes

CONDITION OF THE MOTHER AFTER DELIVERY

Temperature:

Pulse:

Blood pressure:

Fundal height :

Uterus : Hard/soft

Vaginal bleeding: Normal/abnormal

CLINICAL CHART OF PUERPERIUM

Date														
Temperature	M	E	M	E	M	E	M	E	M	E	M	E	M	E
Pulse														
Respiration														
Fundal Height														
Lochia														
Urine														
Motion														

CONDITION OF MOTHER /BABY ON DISCHARGE

Date			
Mother		Baby	
General condition		General condition	
Uterus		Weight	
Lochia		Length	
Episiotomy		Head circumference	
Breast		Chest circumference	
		Feeds	
		Urine/stool	
		Date of cord separation	

INSTRUCTION ON DISCHARGE

CONDUCT OF NORMAL DELIVERY

Name:

Age:

Hospital no:

Date of admission:

Date of delivery:

Prenatal record

Gravida:

PARA:

LMP:

EDD:

ANTENATAL ATTENDANCE

Date	Weight	Urine		BP	Fundal Height	Gestational Age	FHR
		Alb.	Sugar				

INVESTIGATIONS /EXAMINATIONS

Blood group:

Hb:

Breasts:

Nipples:

General conditions:

OBSTETRICAL HISTORY

S. No.	Date	Abortion	Preterm	Fullterm	Type of Delivery	Sex	Alive/Stillbirth

I Year

ADMISSION TO LABOR ROOM

Admission on------------------------------at------------------------am/pm.

Period of gestation:

Contraction commenced on--------------------at-------------am/pm.

Height of fundus:

Presentation:

Position:

Head: Engaged /not engaged

Nature of contraction:

FHR:

Bladder:

Bowel:

Vaginal examination

Effacement:

Cervix dilatation:

Station:

Membranes: Intact/ruptured on

Liquor:

DELIVERY NOTES

Membranes ruptured at ------------am/pm, on--------------------------------

Spontaneously/artificially

Reason:

Expulsive contraction commenced at --------am/pm, on-------------baby.

Born at----------am/pm, on ----------------------

Sex of the baby:

Apgar Score:

Condition of baby at birth

Active/limp/asphyxiated

Alive/stillborn/macerated

Cause:

TREATMENT AT BIRTH

PLACENTA /MEMBRANES

Delivered at-----------am/pm, on ------------------------

Spontaneously /helped/manually removed

Type of placenta; healthy/infarcts

Maternal side: Complete/Incomplete

Fetal side:

Weight:

Cord insertion:

Cord length:

BLOOD LOSS

Before delivery of placenta ---------------

During delivery of placenta ---------------

After delivery of placenta ---------------

Total ---------------

CONDITION OF PERINEUM

Intact/episiotomy

Torn/degree

Repaired with

DRUGS GIVEN DURING DELIVERY

DRUGS GIVEN AFTER DELIVERY

LABOR SUMMARY

Type of labor:

Mode of delivery :

Length of labor

I stage of labor ---------------hours ------------minutes

II stage of labor ---------------hours ------------minutes

III stage of labor ---------------hours ------------minutes

Total ---------------hours ------------minutes

CONDITION OF THE MOTHER AFTER DELIVERY

Temperature:

Pulse:

Blood pressure:

Fundal height :

Uterus: Hard/soft

Vaginal bleeding: Normal/abnormal

CLINICAL CHART OF PUERPERIUM

Date														
Temperature	M	E	M	E	M	E	M	E	M	E	M	E	M	E
Pulse														
Respiration														
Fundal Height														
Lochia														
Urine														
Motion														

CONDITION OF MOTHER /BABY ON DISCHARGE

Date			
Mother		Baby	
General condition		General condition	
Uterus		Weight	
Lochia		Length	
Episiotomy		Head circumference	
Breast		Chest circumference	
		Feeds	
		Urine/stool	
		Date of cord separation	

INSTRUCTION ON DISCHARGE

CONDUCT OF NORMAL DELIVERY

Name:

Age:

Hospital no:

Date of admission:

Date of delivery:

Prenatal record

Gravida:

PARA:

LMP:

EDD:

ANTENATAL ATTENDANCE

Date	Weight	Urine		BP	Fundal Height	Gestational Age	FHR
		Alb.	Sugar				

INVESTIGATIONS /EXAMINATIONS

Blood group:

Hb:

Breasts:

Nipples:

General conditions:

OBSTETRICAL HISTORY

S. No.	Date	Abortion	Preterm	Fullterm	Type of Delivery	Sex	Alive/Stillbirth

I Year

ADMISSION TO LABOR ROOM

Admission on-----------------------------at------------------------am/pm.

Period of gestation:

Contraction commenced on-------------------at-------------am/pm.

Height of fundus:

Presentation:

Position:

Head: Engaged/not engaged

Nature of contraction:

FHR:

Bladder:

Bowel:

Vaginal examination

Effacement:

Cervix dilatation:

Station:

Membranes: Intact/ruptured on

Liquor:

DELIVERY NOTES

Membranes ruptured at ------------am/pm, on---------------------------------

Spontaneously/artificially

Reason:

Expulsive contraction commenced at --------am/pm, on------------baby.

Born at----------am/pm, on -----------------------

Sex of the baby:

Apgar Score:

Condition of baby at birth

Active/limp/asphyxiated

Alive/stillborn/macerated

Cause:

TREATMENT AT BIRTH

PLACENTA /MEMBRANES

Delivered at-----------am/pm, on ------------------------

Spontaneously/helped/manually removed

Type of placenta; healthy/infarcts

Maternal side: Complete/incomplete

Fetal side:

Weight:

Cord insertion:

Cord length:

BLOOD LOSS

Before delivery of placenta ----------------

During delivery of placenta ----------------

After delivery of placenta ----------------

Total ----------------

CONDITION OF PERINEUM

Intact/episiotomy

Torn/degree

Repaired with

DRUGS GIVEN DURING DELIVERY

DRUGS GIVEN AFTER DELIVERY

LABOR SUMMARY

Type of labor:

Mode of delivery:

Length of labor

I stage of labor ---------------hours ------------minutes

II stage of labor ---------------hours ------------minutes

III stage of labor ---------------hours ------------minutes

Total ---------------hours ------------minutes

CONDITION OF THE MOTHER AFTER DELIVERY

Temperature:

Pulse:

Blood pressure:

Fundal height:

Uterus: Hard/soft

Vaginal bleeding: Normal/abnormal

CLINICAL CHART OF PUERPERIUM

Date														
Temperature	M	E	M	E	M	E	M	E	M	E	M	E	M	E
Pulse														
Respiration														
Fundal Height														
Lochia														
Urine														
Motion														

CONDITION OF MOTHER /BABY ON DISCHARGE

Date			
Mother		Baby	
General condition		General condition	
Uterus		Weight	
Lochia		Length	
Episiotomy		Head circumference	
Breast		Chest circumference	
		Feeds	
		Urine/stool	
		Date of cord separation	

INSTRUCTION ON DISCHARGE

I Year

CONDUCT OF NORMAL DELIVERY

Name:

Age:

Hospital no:

Date of admission:

Date of delivery:

Prenatal record

Gravida:

PARA:

LMP:

EDD:

ANTENATAL ATTENDANCE

Date	Weight	Urine		BP	Fundal Height	Gestational Age	FHR
		Alb.	Sugar				

INVESTIGATIONS/EXAMINATIONS

Blood group:

Hb:

Breasts:

Nipples:

General conditions:

OBSTETRICAL HISTORY

S. No.	Date	Abortion	Preterm	Fullterm	Type of Delivery	Sex	Alive/Stillbirth

ADMISSION TO LABOR ROOM

Admission on-----------------------------at-------------------------am/pm.

Period of gestation:

Contraction commenced on-------------------at-------------am/pm.

Height of fundus:

Presentation:

Position:

Head: Engaged/not engaged

Nature of contraction:

FHR:

Bladder:

Bowel:

Vaginal examination

Effacement:

Cervix dilatation:

Station:

Membranes: Intact/ruptured on

Liquor:

DELIVERY NOTES

Membranes ruptured at ------------am/pm, on--------------------------------

Spontaneously/artificially

Reason:

Expulsive contraction commenced at --------am/pm, on-------------baby.

Born at----------am/pm, on ----------------------

Sex of the baby:

Apgar Score:

Condition of baby at birth

Active/limp/asphyxiated

Alive/stillborn/macerated

Cause:

TREATMENT AT BIRTH

PLACENTA /MEMBRANES

Delivered at-----------am/pm, on ------------------------

Spontaneously/helped/manually removed

Type of placenta; healthy/infarcts

Maternal side: Complete/incomplete

Fetal side:

Weight:

Cord insertion:

Cord length:

BLOOD LOSS

Before delivery of placenta ---------------

During delivery of placenta ---------------

After delivery of placenta ---------------

Total ---------------

CONDITION OF PERINEUM

Intact/episiotomy

Torn/degree

Repaired with

DRUGS GIVEN DURING DELIVERY

DRUGS GIVEN AFTER DELIVERY

LABOR SUMMARY

Type of labor:

Mode of delivery:

Length of labor

I stage of labor ---------------hours ------------minutes

II stage of labor ---------------hours ------------minutes

III stage of labor ---------------hours ------------minutes

Total ---------------hours-------------minutes

CONDITION OF THE MOTHER AFTER DELIVERY

Temperature:

Pulse:

Blood pressure:

Fundal height:

Uterus: Hard/soft

Vaginal bleeding: Normal/abnormal

CLINICAL CHART OF PUERPERIUM

Date														
Temperature	M	E	M	E	M	E	M	E	M	E	M	E	M	E
Pulse														
Respiration														
Fundal Height														
Lochia														
Urine														
Motion														

CONDITION OF MOTHER /BABY ON DISCHARGE

Date			
Mother		Baby	
General condition		General condition	
Uterus		Weight	
Lochia		Length	
Episiotomy		Head circumference	
Breast		Chest circumference	
		Feeds	
		Urine/stool	
		Date of cord separation	

INSTRUCTION ON DISCHARGE

CONDUCT OF NORMAL DELIVERY

Name:

Age:

Hospital no:

Date of admission:

Date of delivery:

Prenatal record

Gravida:

PARA:

LMP:

EDD:

ANTENATAL ATTENDANCE

Date	Weight	Urine		BP	Fundal Height	Gestational Age	FHR
		Alb.	Sugar				

INVESTIGATIONS /EXAMINATIONS

Blood group:

Hb:

Breasts:

Nipples:

General conditions:

OBSTETRICAL HISTORY

S. No.	Date	Abortion	Preterm	Fullterm	Type of Delivery	Sex	Alive/Stillbirth

I Year

ADMISSION TO LABOR ROOM

Admission on------------------------------at------------------------am/pm.

Period of gestation:

Contraction commenced on-------------------at--------------am/pm.

Height of fundus:

Presentation:

Position:

Head: Engaged /not engaged

Nature of contraction:

FHR:

Bladder:

Bowel:

Vaginal examination

Effacement:

Cervix dilatation:

Station:

Membranes: Intact/ruptured on

Liquor:

DELIVERY NOTES

Membranes ruptured at ------------am/pm, on---------------------------------

Spontaneously/artificially

Reason:

Expulsive contraction commenced at --------am/pm, on-------------baby.

Born at---------am/pm, on -----------------------

Sex of the baby:

Apgar Score:

Condition of baby at birth

Active/limp/asphyxiated

Alive/stillborn/macerated

Cause:

TREATMENT AT BIRTH

PLACENTA /MEMBRANES

Delivered at-----------am/pm, on ------------------------

Spontaneously /helped/manually removed

Type of placenta; healthy/infarcts

Maternal side: Complete/incomplete

Fetal side:

Weight:

Cord insertion:

Cord length:

BLOOD LOSS

Before delivery of placenta	----------------
During delivery of placenta	----------------
After delivery of placenta	----------------
Total	----------------

CONDITION OF PERINEUM

Intact/episiotomy

Torn/degree

Repaired with

DRUGS GIVEN DURING DELIVERY

DRUGS GIVEN AFTER DELIVERY

LABOR SUMMARY

Type of labor:

Mode of delivery :

Length of labor

I stage of labor	---------------hours ------------minutes
II stage of labor	---------------hours ------------minutes
III stage of labor	---------------hours ------------minutes
Total	---------------hours ------------minutes

CONDITION OF THE MOTHER AFTER DELIVERY

Temperature:

Pulse:

Blood pressure:

Fundal height:

Uterus: Hard/soft

Vaginal bleeding: Normal/abnormal

CLINICAL CHART OF PUERPERIUM

Date														
Temperature	M	E	M	E	M	E	M	E	M	E	M	E	M	E
Pulse														
Respiration														
Fundal Height														
Lochia														
Urine														
Motion														

CONDITION OF MOTHER /BABY ON DISCHARGE

Date			
Mother		Baby	
General condition		General condition	
Uterus		Weight	
Lochia		Length	
Episiotomy		Head circumference	
Breast		Chest circumference	
		Feeds	
		Urine/stool	
		Date of cord separation	

INSTRUCTION ON DISCHARGE

CONDUCT OF NORMAL DELIVERY

Name:

Age:

Hospital no:

Date of admission:

Date of delivery:

Prenatal record

Gravida:

PARA:

LMP:

EDD:

ANTENATAL ATTENDANCE

Date	Weight	Urine		BP	Fundal Height	Gestational Age	FHR
		Alb.	Sugar				

INVESTIGATIONS /EXAMINATIONS

Blood group:

Hb:

Breasts:

Nipples:

General conditions:

OBSTETRICAL HISTORY

S. No.	Date	Abortion	Preterm	Fullterm	Type of Delivery	Sex	Alive/Stillbirth

I Year

ADMISSION TO LABOR ROOM

Admission on-------------------------------at--------------------------am/pm.

Period of gestation:

Contraction commenced on--------------------at--------------am/pm.

Height of fundus:

Presentation:

Position:

Head: Engaged /not engaged

Nature of contraction:

FHR:

Bladder:

Bowel:

Vaginal examination

Effacement:

Cervix dilatation:

Station:

Membranes: Intact/ruptured on

Liquor:

DELIVERY NOTES

Membranes ruptured at ------------am/pm, on--------------------------------

Spontaneously/artificially

Reason:

Expulsive contraction commenced at --------am/pm, on------------baby.

Born at---------am/pm, on ----------------------

Sex of the baby:

Apgar Score:

Condition of baby at birth

Active/limp/asphyxiated

Alive/stillborn/macerated

Cause:

TREATMENT AT BIRTH

PLACENTA /MEMBRANES

Delivered at-----------am/pm, on -------------------------

Spontaneously /helped/manually removed

Type of placenta; healthy/infarcts

Maternal side: Complete/incomplete

Fetal side:

Weight:

Cord insertion:

Cord length:

BLOOD LOSS

Before delivery of placenta ----------------

During delivery of placenta ----------------

After delivery of placenta ----------------

Total ----------------

CONDITION OF PERINEUM

Intact/episiotomy

Torn/degree

Repaired with

DRUGS GIVEN DURING DELIVERY

DRUGS GIVEN AFTER DELIVERY

LABOR SUMMARY

Type of labor:

Mode of delivery:

Length of labor

I stage of labor ---------------hours ------------minutes

II stage of labor ---------------hours ------------minutes

III stage of labor ---------------hours ------------minutes

Total ---------------hours ------------minutes

CONDITION OF THE MOTHER AFTER DELIVERY

Temperature:

Pulse:

Blood pressure:

Fundal height:

Uterus: Hard/soft

Vaginal bleeding: Normal/abnormal

CLINICAL CHART OF PUERPERIUM

Date														
Temperature	M	E	M	E	M	E	M	E	M	E	M	E	M	E
Pulse														
Respiration														
Fundal Height														
Lochia														
Urine														
Motion														

CONDITION OF MOTHER /BABY ON DISCHARGE

Date			
Mother		Baby	
General condition		General condition	
Uterus		Weight	
Lochia		Length	
Episiotomy		Head circumference	
Breast		Chest circumference	
		Feeds	
		Urine/stool	
		Date of cord separation	

INSTRUCTION ON DISCHARGE

CONDUCT OF NORMAL DELIVERY

Name:

Age:

Hospital no:

Date of admission:

Date of delivery:

Prenatal record

Gravida:

PARA:

LMP:

EDD:

ANTENATAL ATTENDANCE

Date	Weight	Urine		BP	Fundal Height	Gestational Age	FHR
		Alb.	Sugar				

INVESTIGATIONS /EXAMINATIONS

Blood group:

Hb:

Breasts:

Nipples:

General conditions:

OBSTETRICAL HISTORY

S. No.	Date	Abortion	Preterm	Fullterm	Type of Delivery	Sex	Alive/Stillbirth

I Year

ADMISSION TO LABOR ROOM

Admission on-----------------------------at-------------------------am/pm.

Period of gestation:

Contraction commenced on--------------------at--------------am/pm.

Height of fundus:

Presentation:

Position:

Head: Engaged/not engaged

Nature of contraction:

FHR:

Bladder:

Bowel:

Vaginal examination

Effacement:

Cervix dilatation:

Station:

Membranes: Intact/ruptured on

Liquor:

DELIVERY NOTES

Membranes ruptured at -----------am/pm, on--------------------------------

Spontaneously/artificially

Reason:

Expulsive contraction commenced at --------am/pm, on------------baby.

Born at---------am/pm, on ---------------------

Sex of the baby:

Apgar Score:

Condition of baby at birth

Active/limp/asphyxiated

Alive/stillborn/macerated

Cause:

TREATMENT AT BIRTH

PLACENTA /MEMBRANES

Delivered at-----------am/pm, on ------------------------

Spontaneously/helped/manually removed

Type of placenta; healthy/infarcts

Maternal side: Complete/incomplete

Fetal side:

Weight:

Cord insertion:

Cord length:

BLOOD LOSS

Before delivery of placenta ----------------

During delivery of placenta ----------------

After delivery of placenta ----------------

Total ----------------

CONDITION OF PERINEUM

Intact/episiotomy

Torn/degree

Repaired with

DRUGS GIVEN DURING DELIVERY

DRUGS GIVEN AFTER DELIVERY

LABOR SUMMARY

Type of labor:

Mode of delivery:

Length of labor

I stage of labor ---------------hours ------------minutes

II stage of labor ---------------hours ------------minutes

III stage of labor ---------------hours ------------minutes

Total ---------------hours ------------minutes

CONDITION OF THE MOTHER AFTER DELIVERY

Temperature:

Pulse:

Blood pressure:

Fundal height:

Uterus: Hard/soft

Vaginal bleeding: Normal/abnormal

CLINICAL CHART OF PUERPERIUM

Date														
Temperature	M	E	M	E	M	E	M	E	M	E	M	E	M	E
Pulse														
Respiration														
Fundal Height														
Lochia														
Urine														
Motion														

CONDITION OF MOTHER /BABY ON DISCHARGE

Date			
Mother		Baby	
General condition		General condition	
Uterus		Weight	
Lochia		Length	
Episiotomy		Head circumference	
Breast		Chest circumference	
		Feeds	
		Urine/stool	
		Date of cord separation	

INSTRUCTION ON DISCHARGE

Name:

Age:

Hospital no:

Date of admission:

Date of delivery:

Prenatal record

Gravida:

PARA:

LMP:

EDD:

ANTENATAL ATTENDANCE

Date	Weight	Urine		BP	Fundal Height	Gestational Age	FHR
		Alb.	Sugar				

INVESTIGATIONS /EXAMINATIONS

Blood group:

Hb:

Breasts:

Nipples:

General conditions:

OBSTETRICAL HISTORY

S. No.	Date	Abortion	Preterm	Fullterm	Type of Delivery	Sex	Alive/Stillbirth

I Year

ADMISSION TO LABOR ROOM

Admission on-----------------------------at-------------------------am/pm.

Period of gestation:

Contraction commenced on--------------------at--------------am/pm.

Height of fundus:

Presentation:

Position:

Head: Engaged/not engaged

Nature of contraction:

FHR:

Bladder:

Bowel:

Vaginal examination

Effacement:

Cervix dilatation:

Station:

Membranes: Intact/ruptured on

Liquor:

DELIVERY NOTES

Membranes ruptured at ------------am/pm, on---------------------------------

Spontaneously/artificially

Reason:

Expulsive contraction commenced at --------am/pm, on-------------baby.

Born at---------am/pm, on ----------------------

Sex of the baby:

Apgar Score:

Condition of baby at birth

Active/limp/asphyxiated

Alive/stillborn/macerated

Cause:

TREATMENT AT BIRTH

PLACENTA /MEMBRANES

Delivered at------------am/pm, on -------------------------

Spontaneously /helped/manually removed

Type of placenta; healthy/infarcts

Maternal side: Complete/incomplete

Fetal side:

Weight:

Cord insertion:

Cord length:

BLOOD LOSS

Before delivery of placenta ----------------

During delivery of placenta ----------------

After delivery of placenta ----------------

Total ----------------

CONDITION OF PERINEUM

Intact/episiotomy

Torn/degree

Repaired with:

DRUGS GIVEN DURING DELIVERY

DRUGS GIVEN AFTER DELIVERY

LABOR SUMMARY

Type of labor:

Mode of delivery:

Length of labor

I stage of labor ---------------hours ------------minutes

II stage of labor ---------------hours ------------minutes

III stage of labor ---------------hours ------------minutes

Total ---------------hours ------------minutes

CONDITION OF THE MOTHER AFTER DELIVERY

Temperature:

Pulse:

Blood pressure:

Fundal height:

Uterus: Hard/soft

Vaginal bleeding: Normal/abnormal

CLINICAL CHART OF PUERPERIUM

Date														
Temperature	M	E	M	E	M	E	M	E	M	E	M	E	M	E
Pulse														
Respiration														
Fundal Height														
Lochia														
Urine														
Motion														

CONDITION OF MOTHER /BABY ON DISCHARGE

Date			
Mother		Baby	
General condition		General condition	
Uterus		Weight	
Lochia		Length	
Episiotomy		Head circumference	
Breast		Chest circumference	
		Feeds	
		Urine/stool	
		Date of cord separation	

I Year

INSTRUCTION ON DISCHARGE

CONDUCT OF NORMAL DELIVERY

Name:

Age:

Hospital no:

Date of admission:

Date of delivery:

Prenatal record

Gravida:

PARA:

LMP:

EDD:

ANTENATAL ATTENDANCE

Date	Weight	Urine		BP	Fundal Height	Gestational Age	FHR
		Alb.	Sugar				

INVESTIGATIONS /EXAMINATIONS

Blood group:

Hb:

Breasts:

Nipples:

General conditions:

OBSTETRICAL HISTORY

S. No.	Date	Abortion	Preterm	Fullterm	Type of Delivery	Sex	Alive/Stillbirth

I Year

ADMISSION TO LABOR ROOM

Admission on------------------------------at-------------------------am/pm.

Period of gestation:

Contraction commenced on--------------------at--------------am/pm.

Height of fundus:

Presentation:

Position:

Head: Engaged/not engaged

Nature of contraction:

FHR:

Bladder:

Bowel:

Vaginal examination

Effacement:

Cervix dilatation:

Station:

Membranes: Intact/ruptured on

Liquor:

DELIVERY NOTES

Membranes ruptured at ------------am/pm, on--------------------------------

Spontaneously/artificially

Reason:

Expulsive contraction commenced at --------am/pm, on------------baby.

Born at---------am/pm, on ----------------------

Sex of the baby:

Apgar Score:

Condition of baby at birth

Active/limp/asphyxiated

Alive/stillborn/macerated

Cause:

TREATMENT AT BIRTH

PLACENTA /MEMBRANES

Delivered at------------am/pm, on -------------------------

Spontaneously/helped/manually removed

Type of placenta; healthy/infarcts

Maternal side: Complete/incomplete

Fetal side:

Weight:

Cord insertion:

Cord length:

BLOOD LOSS

Before delivery of placenta -----------------

During delivery of placenta -----------------

After delivery of placenta -----------------

Total -----------------

CONDITION OF PERINEUM

Intact/episiotomy

Torn/degree

Repaired with

DRUGS GIVEN DURING DELIVERY

DRUGS GIVEN AFTER DELIVERY

LABOR SUMMARY

Type of labor:

Mode of delivery:

Length of labor

I stage of labor ---------------hours ------------minutes

II stage of labor ---------------hours ------------minutes

III stage of labor ---------------hours ------------minutes

Total ---------------hours ------------minutes

CONDITION OF THE MOTHER AFTER DELIVERY

Temperature:

Pulse:

Blood pressure:

Fundal height:

Uterus: Hard/soft

Vaginal bleeding: Normal/abnormal

CLINICAL CHART OF PUERPERIUM

Date														
Temperature	M	E	M	E	M	E	M	E	M	E	M	E	M	E
Pulse														
Respiration														
Fundal Height														
Lochia														
Urine														
Motion														

CONDITION OF MOTHER /BABY ON DISCHARGE

Date			
Mother		Baby	
General condition		General condition	
Uterus		Weight	
Lochia		Length	
Episiotomy		Head circumference	
Breast		Chest circumference	
		Feeds	
		Urine/stool	
		Date of cord separation	

I Year

INSTRUCTION ON DISCHARGE

CONDUCT OF NORMAL DELIVERY

Name:

Age:

Hospital no:

Date of admission:

Date of delivery:

Prenatal record

Gravida:

PARA:

LMP:

EDD:

ANTENATAL ATTENDANCE

Date	Weight	Urine		BP	Fundal Height	Gestational Age	FHR
		Alb.	Sugar				

INVESTIGATIONS/EXAMINATIONS

Blood group:

Hb:

Breasts:

Nipples:

General conditions:

OBSTETRICAL HISTORY

S. No.	Date	Abortion	Preterm	Fullterm	Type of Delivery	Sex	Alive/Stillbirth

ADMISSION TO LABOR ROOM

Admission on-----------------------------at-------------------------am/pm.

Period of gestation:

Contraction commenced on--------------------at--------------am/pm.

Height of fundus:

Presentation:

Position:

Head: Engaged/not engaged

Nature of contraction:

FHR:

Bladder:

Bowel:

Vaginal examination

Effacement:

Cervix dilatation:

Station:

Membranes: Intact/ruptured on

Liquor:

DELIVERY NOTES

Membranes ruptured at ------------am/pm, on---------------------------------

Spontaneously/artificially

Reason:

Expulsive contraction commenced at --------am/pm, on-------------baby.

Born at----------am/pm, on -----------------------

Sex of the baby:

Apgar Score:

Condition of baby at birth

Active/limp/asphyxiated

Alive/stillborn/macerated

Cause:

TREATMENT AT BIRTH

PLACENTA /MEMBRANES

Delivered at-----------am/pm, on -----------------------

Spontaneously /helped/manually removed

Type of placenta; healthy/infarcts

Maternal side: Complete/incomplete

Fetal side:

Weight:

Cord insertion:

Cord length:

BLOOD LOSS

Before delivery of placenta ----------------

During delivery of placenta ----------------

After delivery of placenta ----------------

Total ----------------

CONDITION OF PERINEUM

Intact/episiotomy

Torn/degree

Repaired with

DRUGS GIVEN DURING DELIVERY

DRUGS GIVEN AFTER DELIVERY

LABOR SUMMARY

Type of labor:

Mode of delivery:

Length of labor

I stage of labor ---------------hours ------------minutes

II stage of labor ---------------hours ------------minutes

III stage of labor ---------------hours ------------minutes

Total ---------------hours ------------minutes

CONDITION OF THE MOTHER AFTER DELIVERY

Temperature:

Pulse:

Blood pressure:

Fundal height:

Uterus: Hard/soft

Vaginal bleeding: Normal/abnormal

CLINICAL CHART OF PUERPERIUM

Date														
Temperature	M	E	M	E	M	E	M	E	M	E	M	E	M	E
Pulse														
Respiration														
Fundal Height														
Lochia														
Urine														
Motion														

CONDITION OF MOTHER /BABY ON DISCHARGE

Date			
Mother		Baby	
General condition		General condition	
Uterus		Weight	
Lochia		Length	
Episiotomy		Head circumference	
Breast		Chest circumference	
		Feeds	
		Urine/stool	
		Date of cord separation	

I Year

INSTRUCTION ON DISCHARGE

Name:

Age:

Hospital no:

Date of admission:

Date of delivery:

Prenatal record

Gravida:

PARA:

LMP:

EDD:

ANTENATAL ATTENDANCE

Date	Weight	Urine		BP	Fundal Height	Gestational Age	FHR
		Alb.	Sugar				

INVESTIGATIONS /EXAMINATIONS

Blood group:

Hb:

Breasts:

Nipples:

General conditions:

OBSTETRICAL HISTORY

S. No.	Date	Abortion	Preterm	Fullterm	Type of Delivery	Sex	Alive/Stillbirth

ADMISSION TO LABOR ROOM

Admission on------------------------------at-------------------------am/pm.

Period of gestation:

Contraction commenced on-------------------at--------------am/pm.

Height of fundus:

Presentation:

Position:

Head: Engaged /not engaged

Nature of contraction:

FHR:

Bladder:

Bowel:

Vaginal examination

Effacement:

Cervix dilatation:

Station:

Membranes: Intact/ruptured on

Liquor:

DELIVERY NOTES

Membranes ruptured at ------------am/pm, on--------------------------------

Spontaneously/artificially

Reason:

Expulsive contraction commenced at --------am/pm, on------------baby.

Born at---------am/pm, on ----------------------

Sex of the baby:

Apgar Score:

Condition of baby at birth

Active/limp/asphyxiated

Alive/stillborn/macerated

Cause:

TREATMENT AT BIRTH

PLACENTA /MEMBRANES

Delivered at------------am/pm, on -------------------------

Spontaneously /helped/manually removed

Type of placenta; healthy/infarcts

Maternal side: Complete/incomplete

Fetal side:

Weight:

Cord insertion:

Cord length:

BLOOD LOSS

Before delivery of placenta -----------------

During delivery of placenta ----------------

After delivery of placenta ----------------

Total ----------------

CONDITION OF PERINEUM

Intact/episiotomy

Torn/degree

Repaired with

DRUGS GIVEN DURING DELIVERY

DRUGS GIVEN AFTER DELIVERY

LABOR SUMMARY

Type of labor:

Mode of delivery:

Length of labor

I stage of labor ---------------hours ------------minutes

II stage of labor ---------------hours ------------minutes

III stage of labor ---------------hours ------------minutes

Total ---------------hours ------------minutes

CONDITION OF THE MOTHER AFTER DELIVERY

Temperature:

Pulse:

Blood pressure:

Fundal height:

Uterus: Hard/soft

Vaginal bleeding: Normal/abnormal

CLINICAL CHART OF PUERPERIUM

Date														
Temperature	M	E	M	E	M	E	M	E	M	E	M	E	M	E
Pulse														
Respiration														
Fundal Height														
Lochia														
Urine														
Motion														

CONDITION OF MOTHER /BABY ON DISCHARGE

Date			
Mother		Baby	
General condition		General condition	
Uterus		Weight	
Lochia		Length	
Episiotomy		Head circumference	
Breast		Chest circumference	
		Feeds	
		Urine/stool	
		Date of cord separation	

INSTRUCTION ON DISCHARGE

CONDUCT OF NORMAL DELIVERY

Name:

Age:

Hospital no:

Date of admission:

Date of delivery:

Prenatal record

Gravida:

PARA:

LMP:

EDD:

ANTENATAL ATTENDANCE

Date	Weight	Urine		BP	Fundal Height	Gestational Age	FHR
		Alb.	Sugar				

INVESTIGATIONS /EXAMINATIONS

Blood group:

Hb:

Breasts:

Nipples:

General conditions:

OBSTETRICAL HISTORY

S. No.	Date	Abortion	Preterm	Fullterm	Type of Delivery	Sex	Alive/Stillbirth

ADMISSION TO LABOR ROOM

Admission on-----------------------------at-------------------------am/pm.

Period of gestation:

Contraction commenced on--------------------at--------------am/pm.

Height of fundus:

Presentation:

Position:

Head: Engaged/not engaged

Nature of contraction:

FHR:

Bladder:

Bowel:

Vaginal examination

Effacement:

Cervix dilatation:

Station:

Membranes: Intact/ruptured on

Liquor:

DELIVERY NOTES

Membranes ruptured at -----------am/pm, on-------------------------------

Spontaneously/artificially

Reason:

Expulsive contraction commenced at --------am/pm, on------------baby.

Born at---------am/pm, on ---------------------

Sex of the baby:

Apgar Score:

Condition of baby at birth

Active/limp/asphyxiated

Alive/stillborn/macerated

Cause:

TREATMENT AT BIRTH

PLACENTA /MEMBRANES

Delivered at------------am/pm, on -------------------------

Spontaneously/helped/manually removed

Type of placenta; healthy/infarcts

Maternal side: Complete/incomplete

Fetal side:

Weight:

Cord insertion:

Cord length:

BLOOD LOSS

Before delivery of placenta	----------------
During delivery of placenta	----------------
After delivery of placenta	----------------
Total	----------------

CONDITION OF PERINEUM

Intact/episiotomy

Torn/degree

Repaired with

DRUGS GIVEN DURING DELIVERY

DRUGS GIVEN AFTER DELIVERY

LABOR SUMMARY

Type of labor:

Mode of delivery:

Length of labor

I stage of labor --------------hours ------------minutes

II stage of labor --------------hours ------------minutes

III stage of labor --------------hours ------------minutes

Total --------------hours ------------minutes

CONDITION OF THE MOTHER AFTER DELIVERY

Temperature:

Pulse:

Blood pressure:

Fundal height:

Uterus: Hard/soft

Vaginal bleeding: Normal/abnormal

CLINICAL CHART OF PUERPERIUM

Date														
Temperature	M	E	M	E	M	E	M	E	M	E	M	E	M	E
Pulse														
Respiration														
Fundal Height														
Lochia														
Urine														
Motion														

CONDITION OF MOTHER /BABY ON DISCHARGE

Date			
Mother		Baby	
General condition		General condition	
Uterus		Weight	
Lochia		Length	
Episiotomy		Head circumference	
Breast		Chest circumference	
		Feeds	
		Urine/stool	
		Date of cord separation	

INSTRUCTION ON DISCHARGE

Name:

Age:

Hospital no:

Date of admission:

Date of delivery:

Prenatal record

Gravida:

PARA:

LMP:

EDD:

ANTENATAL ATTENDANCE

Date	Weight	Urine		BP	Fundal Height	Gestational Age	FHR
		Alb.	Sugar				

INVESTIGATIONS/EXAMINATIONS

Blood group:

Hb:

Breasts:

Nipples:

General conditions:

OBSTETRICAL HISTORY

S. No.	Date	Abortion	Preterm	Fullterm	Type of Delivery	Sex	Alive/Stillbirth

ADMISSION TO LABOR ROOM

Admission on-------------------------------at--------------------------am/pm.

Period of gestation:

Contraction commenced on--------------------at--------------am/pm.

Height of fundus:

Presentation:

Position:

Head: Engaged/not engaged

Nature of contraction:

FHR:

Bladder:

Bowel:

Vaginal examination

Effacement:

Cervix dilatation:

Station:

Membranes: Intact/ruptured on

Liquor:

DELIVERY NOTES

Membranes ruptured at ------------am/pm, on--------------------------------

Spontaneously/artificially

Reason:

Expulsive contraction commenced at --------am/pm, on------------baby.

Born at---------am/pm, on -----------------------

Sex of the baby:

Apgar Score:

Condition of baby at birth

Active/limp/asphyxiated

Alive/stillborn/macerated

Cause:

TREATMENT AT BIRTH

PLACENTA /MEMBRANES

Delivered at------------am/pm, on -------------------------

Spontaneously/helped/manually removed

Type of placenta; healthy/infarcts

Maternal side: Complete/incomplete

Fetal side:

Weight:

Cord insertion:

Cord length:

BLOOD LOSS

Before delivery of placenta	----------------
During delivery of placenta	----------------
After delivery of placenta	----------------
Total	----------------

CONDITION OF PERINEUM

Intact/episiotomy

Torn/degree

Repaired with

DRUGS GIVEN DURING DELIVERY

DRUGS GIVEN AFTER DELIVERY

LABOR SUMMARY

Type of labor:

Mode of delivery:

Length of labor

I stage of labor ---------------hours ------------minutes

II stage of labor ---------------hours ------------minutes

III stage of labor ---------------hours ------------minutes

Total ---------------hours ------------minutes

CONDITION OF THE MOTHER AFTER DELIVERY

Temperature:

Pulse:

Blood pressure:

Fundal height:

Uterus: Hard/soft

Vaginal bleeding: Normal/abnormal

CLINICAL CHART OF PUERPERIUM

Date														
Temperature	M	E	M	E	M	E	M	E	M	E	M	E	M	E
Pulse														
Respiration														
Fundal Height														
Lochia														
Urine														
Motion														

CONDITION OF MOTHER /BABY ON DISCHARGE

Date			
Mother		Baby	
General condition		General condition	
Uterus		Weight	
Lochia		Length	
Episiotomy		Head circumference	
Breast		Chest circumference	
		Feeds	
		Urine/stool	
		Date of cord separation	

INSTRUCTION ON DISCHARGE

CONDUCT OF NORMAL DELIVERY

Name:

Age:

Hospital no:

Date of admission:

Date of delivery:

Prenatal record

Gravida:

PARA:

LMP:

EDD:

ANTENATAL ATTENDANCE

Date	Weight	Urine		BP	Fundal Height	Gestational Age	FHR
		Alb.	Sugar				

INVESTIGATIONS/EXAMINATIONS

Blood group:

Hb:

Breasts:

Nipples:

General conditions:

OBSTETRICAL HISTORY

S. No.	Date	Abortion	Preterm	Fullterm	Type of Delivery	Sex	Alive/Stillbirth

ADMISSION TO LABOR ROOM

Admission on------------------------------at-------------------------am/pm.

Period of gestation:

Contraction commenced on--------------------at-------------am/pm.

Height of fundus:

Presentation:

Position:

Head: Engaged/not engaged

Nature of contraction:

FHR:

Bladder:

Bowel:

Vaginal examination

Effacement:

Cervix dilatation:

Station:

Membranes: Intact/ruptured on

Liquor:

DELIVERY NOTES

Membranes ruptured at ------------am/pm, on--------------------------------

Spontaneously/artificially

Reason:

Expulsive contraction commenced at --------am/pm, on------------baby.

Born at---------am/pm, on ----------------------

Sex of the baby:

Apgar Score:

Condition of baby at birth

Active/limp/asphyxiated

Alive/stillborn/macerated

Cause:

TREATMENT AT BIRTH

PLACENTA /MEMBRANES

Delivered at------------am/pm, on -------------------------

Spontaneously/helped/manually removed

Type of placenta; healthy/infarcts

Maternal side: Complete/incomplete

Fetal side:

Weight:

Cord insertion:

Cord length:

BLOOD LOSS

Before delivery of placenta ----------------

During delivery of placenta ----------------

After delivery of placenta ----------------

Total ----------------

CONDITION OF PERINEUM

Intact/episiotomy

Torn/degree

Repaired with

DRUGS GIVEN DURING DELIVERY

DRUGS GIVEN AFTER DELIVERY

LABOR SUMMARY

Type of labor:

Mode of delivery:

Length of labor

I stage of labor ---------------hours ------------minutes

II stage of labor ---------------hours ------------minutes

III stage of labor ---------------hours ------------minutes

Total ---------------hours ------------minutes

CONDITION OF THE MOTHER AFTER DELIVERY

Temperature:

Pulse:

Blood pressure:

Fundal height:

Uterus: Hard/soft

Vaginal bleeding: Normal/abnormal

CLINICAL CHART OF PUERPERIUM

Date														
Temperature	M	E	M	E	M	E	M	E	M	E	M	E	M	E
Pulse														
Respiration														
Fundal Height														
Lochia														
Urine														
Motion														

CONDITION OF MOTHER /BABY ON DISCHARGE

Date			
Mother		Baby	
General condition		General condition	
Uterus		Weight	
Lochia		Length	
Episiotomy		Head circumference	
Breast		Chest circumference	
		Feeds	
		Urine/stool	
		Date of cord separation	

INSTRUCTION ON DISCHARGE

I Year

CONDUCT OF NORMAL DELIVERY

Name:

Age:

Hospital no:

Date of admission:

Date of delivery:

Prenatal record

Gravida:

PARA:

LMP:

EDD:

ANTENATAL ATTENDANCE

Date	Weight	Urine		BP	Fundal Height	Gestational Age	FHR
		Alb.	Sugar				

INVESTIGATIONS/EXAMINATIONS

Blood group:

Hb:

Breasts:

Nipples:

General conditions:

OBSTETRICAL HISTORY

S. No.	Date	Abortion	Preterm	Fullterm	Type of Delivery	Sex	Alive/Stillbirth

ADMISSION TO LABOR ROOM

Admission on-----------------------------at-------------------------am/pm.

Period of gestation:

Contraction commenced on--------------------at--------------am/pm.

Height of fundus:

Presentation:

Position:

Head: Engaged /not engaged

Nature of contraction:

FHR:

Bladder:

Bowel:

Vaginal examination

Effacement:

Cervix dilatation:

Station:

Membranes: Intact/ruptured on

Liquor:

DELIVERY NOTES

Membranes ruptured at ------------am/pm, on---------------------------------

Spontaneously/artificially

Reason:

Expulsive contraction commenced at --------am/pm, on-------------baby.

Born at----------am/pm, on ----------------------

Sex of the baby:

Apgar Score:

Condition of baby at birth

Active/limp/asphyxiated

Alive/stillborn/macerated

Cause:

TREATMENT AT BIRTH

PLACENTA /MEMBRANES

Delivered at------------am/pm, on -------------------------

Spontaneously/helped/manually removed

Type of placenta; healthy/infarcts

Maternal side: Complete/incomplete

Fetal side:

Weight:

Cord insertion:

Cord length:

BLOOD LOSS

Before delivery of placenta ----------------

During delivery of placenta ----------------

After delivery of placenta ----------------

Total ----------------

CONDITION OF PERINEUM

Intact/episiotomy

Torn/degree

Repaired with

DRUGS GIVEN DURING DELIVERY

DRUGS GIVEN AFTER DELIVERY

LABOR SUMMARY

Type of labor:

Mode of delivery:

Length of labor

I stage of labor ---------------hours ------------minutes

II stage of labor ---------------hours ------------minutes

III stage of labor ---------------hours ------------minutes

Total ---------------hours ------------minutes

CONDITION OF THE MOTHER AFTER DELIVERY

Temperature:

Pulse:

Blood pressure:

Fundal height:

Uterus: Hard/soft

Vaginal bleeding: Normal/abnormal

CLINICAL CHART OF PUERPERIUM

Date														
Temperature	M	E	M	E	M	E	M	E	M	E	M	E	M	E
Pulse														
Respiration														
Fundal Height														
Lochia														
Urine														
Motion														

CONDITION OF MOTHER /BABY ON DISCHARGE

Date			
Mother		Baby	
General condition		General condition	
Uterus		Weight	
Lochia		Length	
Episiotomy		Head circumference	
Breast		Chest circumference	
		Feeds	
		Urine/stool	
		Date of cord separation	

INSTRUCTION ON DISCHARGE

CONDUCT OF NORMAL DELIVERY

Name:

Age:

Hospital no:

Date of admission:

Date of delivery:

Prenatal record

Gravida:

PARA:

LMP:

EDD:

ANTENATAL ATTENDANCE

Date	Weight	Urine		BP	Fundal Height	Gestational Age	FHR
		Alb.	Sugar				

INVESTIGATIONS /EXAMINATIONS

Blood group:

Hb:

Breasts:

Nipples:

General conditions:

OBSTETRICAL HISTORY

S. No.	Date	Abortion	Preterm	Fullterm	Type of Delivery	Sex	Alive/Stillbirth

ADMISSION TO LABOR ROOM

Admission on------------------------------at-------------------------am/pm.

Period of gestation:

Contraction commenced on-------------------at--------------am/pm.

Height of fundus:

Presentation:

Position:

Head: Engaged/not engaged

Nature of contraction:

FHR:

Bladder:

Bowel:

Vaginal examination

Effacement:

Cervix dilatation:

Station:

Membranes: Intact/ruptured on

Liquor:

DELIVERY NOTES

Membranes ruptured at ------------am/pm, on--------------------------------

Spontaneously/artificially

Reason:

Expulsive contraction commenced at --------am/pm, on-------------baby.

Born at----------am/pm, on ----------------------

Sex of the baby:

Apgar Score:

Condition of baby at birth

Active/limp/asphyxiated

Alive/stillborn/macerated

Cause:

TREATMENT AT BIRTH

PLACENTA /MEMBRANES

Delivered at-----------am/pm, on ------------------------

Spontaneously /helped/manually removed

Type of placenta; healthy/infarcts

Maternal side: Complete/incomplete

Fetal side:

Weight:

Cord insertion:

Cord length:

BLOOD LOSS

Before delivery of placenta ----------------

During delivery of placenta ----------------

After delivery of placenta ----------------

Total ----------------

CONDITION OF PERINEUM

Intact/episiotomy

Torn/degree

Repaired with

DRUGS GIVEN DURING DELIVERY

DRUGS GIVEN AFTER DELIVERY

LABOR SUMMARY

Type of labor

Mode of delivery:

Length of labor

I stage of labor ---------------hours ------------minutes

II stage of labor ---------------hours ------------minutes

III stage of labor ---------------hours ------------minutes

Total ---------------hours ------------minutes

CONDITION OF THE MOTHER AFTER DELIVERY

Temperature:

Pulse:

Blood pressure:

Fundal height:

Uterus: Hard/soft

Vaginal bleeding: Normal/abnormal

CLINICAL CHART OF PUERPERIUM

Date														
Temperature	M	E	M	E	M	E	M	E	M	E	M	E	M	E
Pulse														
Respiration														
Fundal Height														
Lochia														
Urine														
Motion														

CONDITION OF MOTHER /BABY ON DISCHARGE

Date			
Mother		Baby	
General condition		General condition	
Uterus		Weight	
Lochia		Length	
Episiotomy		Head circumference	
Breast		Chest circumference	
		Feeds	
		Urine/stool	
		Date of cord separation	

INSTRUCTION ON DISCHARGE

CONDUCT OF NORMAL DELIVERY

Name:

Age:

Hospital no:

Date of admission:

Date of delivery:

Prenatal record

Gravida:

PARA:

LMP:

EDD:

ANTENATAL ATTENDANCE

Date	Weight	Urine		BP	Fundal Height	Gestational Age	FHR
		Alb.	Sugar				

INVESTIGATIONS/EXAMINATIONS

Blood group:

Hb:

Breasts:

Nipples:

General conditions:

OBSTETRICAL HISTORY

S. No.	Date	Abortion	Preterm	Fullterm	Type of Delivery	Sex	Alive/Stillbirth

I Year

ADMISSION TO LABOR ROOM

Admission on-----------------------------at-------------------------am/pm.

Period of gestation:

Contraction commenced on-------------------at--------------am/pm.

Height of fundus:

Presentation:

Position:

Head: Engaged/not engaged

Nature of contraction:

FHR:

Bladder:

Bowel:

Vaginal examination

Effacement:

Cervix dilatation:

Station:

Membranes: Intact/ruptured on

Liquor:

DELIVERY NOTES

Membranes ruptured at ------------am/pm, on--------------------------------

Spontaneously/artificially

Reason:

Expulsive contraction commenced at --------am/pm, on-------------baby.

Born at----------am/pm, on ----------------------

Sex of the baby:

Apgar Score:

Condition of baby at birth

Active/limp/asphyxiated

Alive/stillborn/macerated

Cause:

TREATMENT AT BIRTH

PLACENTA /MEMBRANES

Delivered at------------am/pm, on -------------------------

Spontaneously/helped/manually removed

Type of placenta; healthy/infarcts

Maternal side: Complete/incomplete

Fetal side:

Weight:

Cord insertion:

Cord length:

BLOOD LOSS

Before delivery of placenta	----------------
During delivery of placenta	----------------
After delivery of placenta	----------------
Total	----------------

CONDITION OF PERINEUM

Intact/episiotomy

Torn/degree

Repaired with

DRUGS GIVEN DURING DELIVERY

DRUGS GIVEN AFTER DELIVERY

LABOR SUMMARY

Type of labor:

Mode of delivery:

Length of labor

I stage of labor	---------------hours ------------minutes
II stage of labor	---------------hours ------------minutes
III stage of labor	---------------hours ------------minutes
Total	---------------hours ------------minutes

CONDITION OF THE MOTHER AFTER DELIVERY

Temperature:

Pulse:

Blood pressure:

Fundal height:

Uterus: Hard /soft

Vaginal bleeding: Normal/abnormal

CLINICAL CHART OF PUERPERIUM

Date														
Temperature	M	E	M	E	M	E	M	E	M	E	M	E	M	E
Pulse														
Respiration														
Fundal Height														
Lochia														
Urine														
Motion														

CONDITION OF MOTHER /BABY ON DISCHARGE

Date			
Mother		Baby	
General condition		General condition	
Uterus		Weight	
Lochia		Length	
Episiotomy		Head circumference	
Breast		Chest circumference	
		Feeds	
		Urine/stool	
		Date of cord separation	

I Year

INSTRUCTION ON DISCHARGE

CONDUCT OF NORMAL DELIVERY

Name:

Age:

Hospital no:

Date of admission:

Date of delivery:

Prenatal record

Gravida:

PARA:

LMP:

EDD:

ANTENATAL ATTENDANCE

Date	Weight	Urine		BP	Fundal Height	Gestational Age	FHR
		Alb.	Sugar				

INVESTIGATIONS /EXAMINATIONS

Blood group:

Hb:

Breasts:

Nipples:

General conditions:

OBSTETRICAL HISTORY

S. No.	Date	Abortion	Preterm	Fullterm	Type of Delivery	Sex	Alive/Stillbirth

ADMISSION TO LABOR ROOM

Admission on-----------------------------at------------------------am/pm.

Period of gestation:

Contraction commenced on-------------------at-------------am/pm.

Height of fundus:

Presentation:

Position:

Head: Engaged /not engaged

Nature of contraction:

FHR:

Bladder:

Bowel:

Vaginal examination

Effacement:

Cervix dilatation:

Station:

Membranes: Intact/ruptured on

Liquor:

DELIVERY NOTES

Membranes ruptured at -----------am/pm, on-------------------------------

Spontaneously/artificially

Reason:

Expulsive contraction commenced at --------am/pm, on------------baby.

Born at----------am/pm, on ----------------------

Sex of the baby:

Apgar Score:

Condition of baby at birth

Active/limp/asphyxiated

Alive/stillborn/macerated

Cause:

TREATMENT AT BIRTH

PLACENTA/MEMBRANES

Delivered at------------am/pm, on --------------------------

Spontaneously/helped/manually removed

Type of placenta; healthy/infarcts

Maternal side: Complete/incomplete

Fetal side:

Weight:

Cord insertion:

Cord length:

BLOOD LOSS

Before delivery of placenta ----------------

During delivery of placenta ----------------

After delivery of placenta ----------------

Total ----------------

CONDITION OF PERINEUM

Intact/episiotomy

Torn/degree

Repaired with

DRUGS GIVEN DURING DELIVERY

DRUGS GIVEN AFTER DELIVERY

LABOR SUMMARY

Type of labor:

Mode of delivery:

Length of labor

I stage of labor ---------------hours ------------minutes

II stage of labor ---------------hours ------------minutes

III stage of labor ---------------hours ------------minutes

Total ---------------hours ------------minutes

CONDITION OF THE MOTHER AFTER DELIVERY

Temperature:

Pulse:

Blood pressure:

Fundal height:

Uterus: Hard/soft

Vaginal bleeding: Normal/abnormal

CLINICAL CHART OF PUERPERIUM

Date														
Temperature	M	E	M	E	M	E	M	E	M	E	M	E	M	E
Pulse														
Respiration														
Fundal Height														
Lochia														
Urine														
Motion														

CONDITION OF MOTHER /BABY ON DISCHARGE

Date			
Mother		Baby	
General condition		General condition	
Uterus		Weight	
Lochia		Length	
Episiotomy		Head circumference	
Breast		Chest circumference	
		Feeds	
		Urine/stool	
		Date of cord separation	

INSTRUCTION ON DISCHARGE

PERFORM EPISIOTOMY AND SUTURING

S. No.	Date	Name of the Mother	Date of Delivery	Age	Indications	Type of Episiotomy	No. of Sutures	Remarks	Nursing Care

PERFORM EPISIOTOMY AND SUTURING

S. No.	Date	Name of the Mother	Date of Delivery	Age	Indications	Type of Episiotomy	No. of Sutures	Remarks	Nursing Care

PERFORM EPISIOTOMY AND SUTURING

S. No.	Date	Name of the Mother	Date of Delivery	Age	Indications	Type of Episiotomy	No. of Sutures	Remarks	Nursing Care

PERFORM EPISIOTOMY AND SUTURING

S. No.	Date	Name of the Mother	Date of Delivery	Age	Indications	Type of Episiotomy	No. of Sutures	Remarks	Nursing Care

PERFORM EPISIOTOMY AND SUTURING

S. No.	Date	Name of the Mother	Date of Delivery	Age	Indications	Type of Episiotomy	No. of Sutures	Remarks	Nursing Care

PERFORM EPISIOTOMY AND SUTURING

S. No.	Date	Name of the Mother	Date of Delivery	Age	Indications	Type of Episiotomy	No. of Sutures	Remarks	Nursing Care

PERFORM EPISIOTOMY AND SUTURING

S. No.	Date	Name of the Mother	Date of Delivery	Age	Indications	Type of Episiotomy	No. of Sutures	Remarks	Nursing Care

PERFORM EPISIOTOMY AND SUTURING

S. No.	Date	Name of the Mother	Date of Delivery	Age	Indications	Type of Episiotomy	No. of Sutures	Remarks	Nursing Care

PERFORM EPISIOTOMY AND SUTURING

S. No.	Date	Name of the Mother	Date of Delivery	Age	Indications	Type of Episiotomy	No. of Sutures	Remarks	Nursing Care

PERFORM EPISIOTOMY AND SUTURING

S. No.	Date	Name of the Mother	Date of Delivery	Age	Indications	Type of Episiotomy	No. of Sutures	Remarks	Nursing Care

INSERTION IUD

S. No.	Date	Name of the Mother	Age	Obstetrical History						Type of IUD	Procedure	Vital Signs	Remarks	Instruction to the Mother
				Abortion	Preterm	Fullterm	Type of Delivery	Sex of Baby	Alive/Stillbirth					

INSERTION IUD

S. No.	Date	Name of the Mother	Age	Obstetrical History						Type of IUD	Procedure	Vital Signs	Remarks	Instruction to the Mother
				Abortion	Preterm	Fullterm	Type of Delivery	Sex of Baby	Alive/Stillbirth					

INSERTION IUD

S. No.	Date	Name of the Mother	Age	Obstetrical History						Type of IUD	Procedure	Vital Signs	Remarks	Instruction to the Mother
				Abortion	Preterm	Fullterm	Type of Delivery	Sex of Baby	Alive/Stillbirth					

INSERTION IUD

S. No.	Date	Name of the Mother	Age	Obstetrical History						Type of IUD	Procedure	Vital Signs	Remarks	Instruction to the Mother
				Abortion	Preterm	Fullterm	Type of Delivery	Sex of Baby	Alive/Stillbirth					

INSERTION IUD

S. No.	Date	Name of the Mother	Age	Obstetrical History						Type of IUD	Procedure	Vital Signs	Remarks	Instruction to the Mother
				Abortion	Preterm	Fullterm	Type of Delivery	Sex of Baby	Alive/Stillbirth					

ANTENATAL CARE PLAN WITH NURSING THEORY APPLICATION

ANTENATAL CARE PLAN

Name of the hospital/maternity center:

Date of care started:

Date of care ended:

PERSONAL HISTORY

Name:

Age:

Date of visit:

Marital status:

Address:

SOCIOECONOMIC HISTORY

Education of the mother:

Education of her husband:

Occupation:

Income:

Religion:

FAMILY HISTORY

Type of family:

No. of persons in the family:

History of any disease in family:

Family tree:

PREVIOUS MEDICAL AND SURGICAL HISTORY

MENSTRUAL HISTORY

OBSTETRICAL HISTORY

Date	Abortion	Preterm	Fullterm	Type of Delivery	Sex	Alive	Wt	Stillbirth	Remarks

ANTENATAL ATTENDANCE

Date	Wt	Urine Alb. Sugar	BP	FHR	Weeks of Gestation	Fundal Ht	Treatment/Remarks

INVESTIGATION

Blood group:

Hb:

VDRL:

Rh:

PHYSICAL EXAMINATION

General Condition

Heart:

Lungs:

Mouth:

Breast and nipples:

Abdomen:

Perineum:

Legs and feet:

Any others if, specify:

Symptoms

Pain:

Appetite:

Heart burn:

Micturition:

Vaginal discharge:

Other:

Obstetrical Examination

Period of gestation:

Presentation:

Position:

Height of fundus:

Head: Engaged/not

Fetal heart rate:

DRUG CHART

S. No.	Name of the Drug	Dose/Route	Action	Indication	Contraindication	Side Effects	Nurses Responsibility

NURSING PROCESS

List of nursing diagnosis:

NURSING CARE PLAN

Assessment	NSG Diagnosis	Objective	Intervention	Implementation	Evaluation

Assessment	NSG Diagnosis	Objective	Intervention	Implementation	Evaluation

NURSING CARE PLAN

Assessment	NSG Diagnosis	Objective	Intervention	Implementation	Evaluation

Assessment	NSG Diagnosis	Objective	Intervention	Implementation	Evaluation

BIBLIOGRAPHY

ANTENATAL CARE PLAN

Name of the hospital/maternity center:

Date of care started:

Date of care ended:

PERSONAL HISTORY

Name:

Age:

Date of visit:

Marital status:

Address:

SOCIOECONOMIC HISTORY

Education of the mother:

Education of her husband:

Occupation:

Income:

Religion:

FAMILY HISTORY

Type of family:

No. of persons in the family:

History of any disease in family:

Family tree:

PREVIOUS MEDICAL AND SURGICAL HISTORY

MENSTRUAL HISTORY

OBSTETRICAL HISTORY

Date	Abortion	Preterm	Fullterm	Type of Delivery	Sex	Alive	Wt	Stillbirth	Remarks

ANTENATAL ATTENDANCE

Date	Wt	Urine Alb. Sugar	BP	FHR	Weeks of Gestation	Fundal Ht	Treatment/Remarks

INVESTIGATION

Blood group:

Hb:

VDRL:

Rh:

PHYSICAL EXAMINATION

General Condition

Heart:

Lungs:

Mouth:

Breast and nipples:

Abdomen:

Perineum:

Legs and feet:

Any others if, specify:

Symptoms

Pain:

Appetite:

Heart burn:

Micturition:

Vaginal discharge:

Other:

Obstetrical Examination

Period of gestation:

Presentation:

Position:

Height of fundus:

Head: Engaged/not

Fetal heart rate:

DRUG CHART

S. No.	Name of the Drug	Dose/Route	Action	Indication	Contraindication	Side Effects	Nurses Responsibility

NURSING PROCESS

List of nursing diagnosis:

THEORY APPLICATION

NURSING CARE PLAN

Assessment	NSG Diagnosis	Objective	Intervention	Implementation	Evaluation

Assessment	NSG Diagnosis	Objective	Intervention	Implementation	Evaluation

NURSING CARE PLAN

Assessment	NSG Diagnosis	Objective	Intervention	Implementation	Evaluation

Assessment	NSG Diagnosis	Objective	Intervention	Implementation	Evaluation

BIBLIOGRAPHY

ANTENATAL CARE PLAN

Name of the hospital/maternity center:

Date of care started:

Date of care ended:

PERSONAL HISTORY

Name:

Age:

Date of visit:

Marital status:

Address:

SOCIOECONOMIC HISTORY

Education of the mother:

Education of her husband:

Occupation:

Income:

Religion:

FAMILY HISTORY

Type of family:

No. of persons in the family:

History of any disease in family:

Family tree:

PREVIOUS MEDICAL AND SURGICAL HISTORY

MENSTRUAL HISTORY

OBSTETRICAL HISTORY

Date	Abortion	Preterm	Fullterm	Type of Delivery	Sex	Alive	Wt	Stillbirth	Remarks

ANTENATAL ATTENDANCE

Date	Wt	Urine Alb. Sugar	BP	FHR	Weeks of Gestation	Fundal Ht	Treatment/Remarks

INVESTIGATION

Blood group:

Hb:

VDRL:

Rh:

PHYSICAL EXAMINATION

General Condition

Heart:

Lungs:

Mouth:

Breast and nipples:

Abdomen:

Perineum:

Legs and feet:

Any others if, specify:

Symptoms

Pain:

Appetite:

Heart burn:

Micturition:

Vaginal discharge:

Other:

Obstetrical Examination

Period of gestation:

Presentation:

Position:

Height of fundus:

Head: Engaged/not

Fetal heart rate:

DRUG CHART

S. No.	Name of the Drug	Dose/Route	Action	Indication	Contraindication	Side Effects	Nurses Responsibility

NURSING PROCESS

List of nursing diagnosis:

THEORY APPLICATION

NURSING CARE PLAN

Assessment	NSG Diagnosis	Objective	Intervention	Implementation	Evaluation

Assessment	NSG Diagnosis	Objective	Intervention	Implementation	Evaluation

NURSING CARE PLAN

Assessment	NSG Diagnosis	Objective	Intervention	Implementation	Evaluation

Assessment	NSG Diagnosis	Objective	Intervention	Implementation	Evaluation

BIBLIOGRAPHY

Name of the hospital/maternity center:

Date of care started:

Date of care ended:

PERSONAL HISTORY

Name:

Age:

Date of visit:

Marital status:

Address:

SOCIOECONOMIC HISTORY

Education of the mother:

Education of her husband:

Occupation:

Income:

Religion:

FAMILY HISTORY

Type of family:

No. of persons in the family:

History of any disease in family:

Family tree:

PREVIOUS MEDICAL AND SURGICAL HISTORY

MENSTRUAL HISTORY

OBSTETRICAL HISTORY

Date	Abortion	Preterm	Fullterm	Type of Delivery	Sex	Alive	Wt	Stillbirth	Remarks

ANTENATAL ATTENDANCE

Date	Wt	Urine Alb. Sugar	BP	FHR	Weeks of Gestation	Fundal Ht	Treatment/Remarks

INVESTIGATION

Blood group:

Hb:

VDRL:

Rh:

PHYSICAL EXAMINATION

General Condition

Heart:

Lungs:

Mouth:

Breast and nipples:

Abdomen:

Perineum:

Legs and feet:

Any others if, specify:

Symptoms

Pain:

Appetite:

Heart burn:

Micturition:

Vaginal discharge:

Other:

Obstetrical Examination

Period of gestation:

Presentation:

Position:

Height of fundus:

Head: Engaged/not

Fetal heart rate:

DRUG CHART

S. No.	Name of the Drug	Dose/Route	Action	Indication	Contraindication	Side Effects	Nurses Responsibility

NURSING PROCESS

List of nursing diagnosis:

NURSING CARE PLAN

Assessment	NSG Diagnosis	Objective	Intervention	Implementation	Evaluation

Assessment	NSG Diagnosis	Objective	Intervention	Implementation	Evaluation

NURSING CARE PLAN

Assessment	NSG Diagnosis	Objective	Intervention	Implementation	Evaluation

Assessment	NSG Diagnosis	Objective	Intervention	Implementation	Evaluation

BIBLIOGRAPHY

Name of the hospital/maternity center:

Date of care started:

Date of care ended:

PERSONAL HISTORY

Name:

Age:

Date of visit:

Marital status:

Address:

SOCIOECONOMIC HISTORY

Education of the mother:

Education of her husband:

Occupation:

Income:

Religion:

FAMILY HISTORY

Type of family:

No. of persons in the family:

History of any disease in family:

Family tree:

PREVIOUS MEDICAL AND SURGICAL HISTORY

MENSTRUAL HISTORY

OBSTETRICAL HISTORY

Date	Abortion	Preterm	Fullterm	Type of Delivery	Sex	Alive	Wt	Stillbirth	Remarks

ANTENATAL ATTENDANCE

Date	Wt	Urine Alb. Sugar	BP	FHR	Weeks of Gestation	Fundal Ht	Treatment/Remarks

INVESTIGATION

Blood group:

Hb:

VDRL:

Rh:

PHYSICAL EXAMINATION

General Condition

Heart:

Lungs:

Mouth:

Breast and nipples:

Abdomen:

Perineum:

Legs and feet:

Any others if, specify:

Symptoms

Pain:

Appetite:

Heart burn:

Micturition:

Vaginal discharge:

Other:

Obstetrical Examination

Period of gestation:

Presentation:

Position:

Height of fundus:

Head: Engaged/not

Fetal heart rate:

DRUG CHART

S. No.	Name of the Drug	Dose/Route	Action	Indication	Contraindication	Side Effects	Nurses Responsibility

NURSING PROCESS

List of nursing diagnosis:

NURSING CARE PLAN

Assessment	NSG Diagnosis	Objective	Intervention	Implementation	Evaluation

Assessment	NSG Diagnosis	Objective	Intervention	Implementation	Evaluation

NURSING CARE PLAN

Assessment	NSG Diagnosis	Objective	Intervention	Implementation	Evaluation

Assessment	NSG Diagnosis	Objective	Intervention	Implementation	Evaluation

BIBLIOGRAPHY

ANTENATAL CARE PLAN

Name of the hospital/maternity center:

Date of care started:

Date of care ended:

PERSONAL HISTORY

Name:

Age:

Date of visit:

Marital status:

Address:

SOCIOECONOMIC HISTORY

Education of the mother:

Education of her husband:

Occupation:

Income:

Religion:

FAMILY HISTORY

Type of family:

No. of persons in the family:

History of any disease in family:

Family tree:

PREVIOUS MEDICAL AND SURGICAL HISTORY

MENSTRUAL HISTORY

OBSTETRICAL HISTORY

Date	Abortion	Preterm	Fullterm	Type of Delivery	Sex	Alive	Wt	Stillbirth	Remarks

ANTENATAL ATTENDANCE

Date	Wt	Urine Alb. Sugar	BP	FHR	Weeks of Gestation	Fundal Ht	Treatment/Remarks

INVESTIGATION

Blood group:

Hb:

VDRL:

Rh:

PHYSICAL EXAMINATION

General Condition

Heart:

Lungs:

Mouth:

Breast and nipples:

Abdomen:

Perineum:

I Year

Legs and feet:

Any others if, specify:

Symptoms

Pain:

Appetite:

Heart burn:

Micturition:

Vaginal discharge:

Other:

Obstetrical Examination

Period of gestation:

Presentation:

Position:

Height of fundus:

Head: Engaged/not

Fetal heart rate:

DRUG CHART

S. No.	Name of the Drug	Dose/Route	Action	Indication	Contraindication	Side Effects	Nurses Responsibility

NURSING PROCESS

List of nursing diagnosis:

THEORY APPLICATION

NURSING CARE PLAN

Assessment	NSG Diagnosis	Objective	Intervention	Implementation	Evaluation

Assessment	NSG Diagnosis	Objective	Intervention	Implementation	Evaluation

NURSING CARE PLAN

Assessment	NSG Diagnosis	Objective	Intervention	Implementation	Evaluation

Assessment	NSG Diagnosis	Objective	Intervention	Implementation	Evaluation

BIBLIOGRAPHY

NATAL CARE PLAN WITH NURSING THEORY APPLICATION

PERSONAL HISTORY

Name:

Age:

Date of visit:

Marital status:

Address:

SOCIOECONOMIC HISTORY

Education of the mother:

Education of her husband:

Occupation:

Income:

Religion:

FAMILY HISTORY

Type of family:

No. of persons in the family:

History of any disease in family:

Family tree:

PREVIOUS MEDICAL AND SURGICAL HISTORY

MENSTRUAL HISTORY

OBSTETRICAL HISTORY

Date	Abortion	Preterm	Fullterm	Type of Delivery	Sex	Alive	Wt	Stillbirth	Remarks

ANTENATAL ATTENDANCE

Date	Wt	Urine Alb. Sugar	BP	FHR	Weeks of Gestation	Fundal Ht	Treatment/Remarks

INVESTIGATION

Blood group:

Hb:

VDRL:

Rh:

ADMISSION TO LABOR ROOM

Admission on:--------------------at---------am/pm.

Contraction commenced on----------------------at-----------am/pm.

Period of gestation:

Membranes: Intact/ruptured on -----------------------at---------am/pm.

Contractions:

Presentation:

Position:

Head engaged/not:

FHR:

Bladder/bowels:

Special observation if, any:

LABOR

Time	BP	Pulse	FHR	Observation	Nursing Care	Intake	Output

DELIVERY RECORD

Membranes ruptured at--------------

Spontaneously/artificially means reason----------------------------

Expulsive contraction commenced at-------------------- on-------------------

DELIVERY OF BABY

Baby born at----------------------- on------------------------------

Sex:

Apgar Score:

Condition at birth: Active/limp/asphyxiated
Stillborn/macerated means cause---------------------

DELIVERY OF PLACENTA AND MEMBRANES

Delivered at------------------- am/pm.

Spontaneously/helped/manually

Type of placenta: Healthy/infarcts----------- %

Complete/incomplete

Weight:

Cord insertion:

Cord length:

BLOOD LOSS

Before delivery of placenta ----------------------------

During delivery of placenta ----------------------------

After delivery of placenta ----------------------------

Total ----------------------------

PERINEUM

Intact/episiotomy Torn/degree

Type of episiotomy:

Repaired with :

DRUG CHART

S. No.	Name of the Drug	Dose/Route	Action	Indication	Contraindication	Side Effects	Nurses Responsibility

LABOR SUMMARY

Type of labor:

Mode of delivery:

Length of labor:

I stage ---------------hours-------------minutes

II stage ---------------hours-------------minutes

III stage ---------------hours-------------minutes

Total ----------------hours-------------minutes

PARTOGRAPH

Patient Name ....
Age ....
Ward ....
Gravida ....
Para ....
Obstetrician ....

Date ....

Time							
Pulse rate							
Temperature							

Fetal Heart Rate	MATERNAL	BLOOD PRESSURE	
			180
			160
			140
			120
			100
			80
			60
			40

Uterine Contractions in 10 Minutes

- <20 Sec
- 20-40 Sec
- >40 Sec

Vaginal Examinations	
Descend	Dilation
-5	10
-4	9
-3	8
-2	7
-1	6
0	5
+1	4
+2	3
+3	2
+4	1
+5	0

Amniotic fluid	
Presentation	
Position of Vertex/Breech	
Effacement	
Caput	
Moulding	
Oxytocin, Units	
Medication	
I.V. Infusion	
Urine	

CONDITION FOLLOWING THE DELIVERY

Temperature:

Pulse:

Respiration:

Fundal height:

Uterus:

Vaginal bleeding:

NURSING PROCESS

List of nursing diagnosis:

NURSING CARE PLAN

Assessment	NSG Diagnosis	Objective	Intervention	Implementation	Evaluation

Assessment	NSG Diagnosis	Objective	Intervention	Implementation	Evaluation

NURSING CARE PLAN

Assessment	NSG Diagnosis	Objective	Intervention	Implementation	Evaluation

Assessment	NSG Diagnosis	Objective	Intervention	Implementation	Evaluation

PERSONAL HISTORY

Name:

Age:

Date of visit:

Marital status:

Address:

SOCIOECONOMIC HISTORY

Education of the mother:

Education of her husband:

Occupation:

Income:

Religion:

FAMILY HISTORY

Type of family:

No. of persons in the family:

History of any disease in family:

Family tree:

PREVIOUS MEDICAL AND SURGICAL HISTORY

MENSTRUAL HISTORY

OBSTETRICAL HISTORY

Date	Abortion	Preterm	Fullterm	Type of Delivery	Sex	Alive	Wt	Stillbirth	Remarks

ANTENATAL ATTENDANCE

Date	Wt	Urine Alb. Sugar	BP	FHR	Weeks of Gestation	Fundal Ht	Treatment/Remarks

INVESTIGATION

Blood group:

Hb:

VDRL:

Rh:

ADMISSION TO LABOR ROOM

Admission on:---------------------at---------am/pm.

Contraction commenced on----------------------at-----------am/pm.

Period of gestation:

Membranes: Intact/ruptured on ----------------------at--------am/pm.

Contractions:

Presentation:

Position:

Head engaged/not:

FHR:

Bladder/bowels:

Special observation if, any:

DELIVERY RECORD

Membranes ruptured at--------------,

Spontaneously/artificially means reason-----------------------------

Expulsive contraction commenced at--------------------- on-------------------

DELIVERY OF BABY

Baby born at----------------------- on------------------------------

Sex:

Apgar Score:

Condition at birth: Active/limp/asphyxiated
Stillborn/macerated means cause----------------------

DELIVERY OF PLACENTA AND MEMBRANES

Delivered at------------------- am/pm.

Spontaneously/helped/manually

Type of placenta: Healthy/infarcts----------- %

Complete/incomplete

Weight:

Cord insertion:

Cord length:

LABOR

Time	BP	Pulse	FHR	Observation	Nursing Care	Intake	Output

BLOOD LOSS

Before delivery of placenta ----------------------------

During delivery of placenta ----------------------------

After delivery of placenta ----------------------------

Total ----------------------------

PERINEUM

Intact/episiotomy Torn/degree

Type of episiotomy:

Repaired with :

DRUG CHART

S. No.	Name of the Drug	Dose/Route	Action	Indication	Contraindication	Side Effects	Nurses Responsibility

LABOR SUMMARY

Type of labor:

Mode of delivery:

Length of labor:

I stage ---------------hours-------------minutes

II stage ---------------hours-------------minutes

III stage --------------hours-------------minutes

Total ---------------hours-------------minutes

CONDITION FOLLOWING THE DELIVERY

Temperature:

Pulse:

Respiration:

Fundal height:

Uterus:

Vaginal bleeding:

PARTOGRAPH

Patient Name ....
Age ....
Ward ....
Gravida ....
Para ....
Obstetrician ....

Date ....

Time														
Pulse rate														
Temperature														

Fetal Heart Rate	MATERNAL	BLOOD PRESSURE																													
			180																												
			160																												
			140																												
			120																												
			100																												
			80																												
			60																												
			40																												

Uterine Contractions in 10 Minutes <20 Sec 20-40 Sec >40 Sec														

Vaginal Examinations															
Descend	Dilation														
-5	10														
-4	9														
-3	8														
-2	7														
-1	6														
0	5														
+1	4														
+2	3														
+3	2														
+4	1														
+5	0														

Amniotic fluid														
Presentation														
Position of Vertex/Breech	○	○	○	○	○	○	○	○	○	○	○	○	○	○
Effacement														
Caput														
Moulding														
Oxytocin, Units														
Medication														
I.V. Infusion														
Urine														

NURSING PROCESS

List of nursing diagnosis:

NURSING CARE PLAN

Assessment	NSG Diagnosis	Objective	Intervention	Implementation	Evaluation

Assessment	NSG Diagnosis	Objective	Intervention	Implementation	Evaluation

NURSING CARE PLAN

Assessment	NSG Diagnosis	Objective	Intervention	Implementation	Evaluation

Assessment	NSG Diagnosis	Objective	Intervention	Implementation	Evaluation

BIBLIOGRAPHY

PERSONAL HISTORY

Name:

Age:

Date of visit:

Marital status:

Address:

SOCIOECONOMIC HISTORY

Education of the mother:

Education of her husband:

Occupation:

Income:

Religion:

FAMILY HISTORY

Type of family:

No. of persons in the family:

History of any disease in family:

Family tree:

PREVIOUS MEDICAL AND SURGICAL HISTORY

MENSTRUAL HISTORY

OBSTETRICAL HISTORY

Date	Abortion	Preterm	Fullterm	Type of Delivery	Sex	Alive	Wt	Stillbirth	Remarks

ANTENATAL ATTENDANCE

Date	Wt	Urine Alb. Sugar	BP	FHR	Weeks of Gestation	Fundal Ht	Treatment/Remarks

INVESTIGATION

Blood group:

Hb:

VDRL:

Rh:

ADMISSION TO LABOR ROOM

Admission on:---------------------at---------am/pm.

Contraction commenced on-----------------------at-----------am/pm.

Period of gestation:

Membranes: Intact/ruptured on ------------------------at--------am/pm.

Contractions:

Presentation:

Position:

Head engaged/not:

FHR:

Bladder/bowels:

Special observation if, any:

LABOR

Time	BP	Pulse	FHR	Observation	Nursing Care	Intake	Output

DELIVERY RECORD

Membranes ruptured at--------------,

Spontaneously/artificially means reason----------------------------

Expulsive contraction commenced at------------------- on-------------------

DELIVERY OF BABY

Baby born at---------------------- on------------------------------

Sex:

Apgar Score:

Condition at birth: Active/limp/asphyxiated
Stillborn/macerated means cause----------------------

DELIVERY OF PLACENTA AND MEMBRANES

Delivered at------------------- am/pm.

Spontaneously/helped/manually

Type of placenta: Healthy/infarcts----------- %

Complete/incomplete

Weight:

Cord insertion:

Cord length:

BLOOD LOSS

Before delivery of placenta -----------------------------

During delivery of placenta -----------------------------

After delivery of placenta -----------------------------

Total -----------------------------

PERINEUM

Intact/episiotomy Torn/degree

Type of episiotomy:

Repaired with :

DRUG CHART

S. No.	Name of the Drug	Dose/Route	Action	Indication	Contraindication	Side Effects	Nurses Responsibility

LABOR SUMMARY

Type of labor:

Mode of delivery:

Length of labor:

I stage ---------------hours-------------minutes

II stage ---------------hours-------------minutes

III stage ---------------hours-------------minutes

Total ----------------hours-------------minutes

PARTOGRAPH

Patient Name ....
Age ....
Ward ....
Gravida ....
Para ....
Obstetrician ....

Date ....

Time														
Pulse rate														
Temperature														

Fetal Heart Rate	MATERNAL	BLOOD PRESSURE													
			180												
			160												
			140												
			120												
			100												
			80												
			60												
			40												

Uterine Contractions in 10 Minutes <20 Sec 20-40 Sec >40 Sec														

Vaginal Examinations															
Descend	Dilation														
-5	10														
-4	9														
-3	8														
-2	7														
-1	6														
0	5														
+1	4														
+2	3														
+3	2														
+4	1														
+5	0														

Amniotic fluid														
Presentation														
Position of Vertex/Breech														
Effacement														
Caput														
Moulding														
Oxytocin, Units														
Medication														
I.V. Infusion														
Urine														

CONDITION FOLLOWING THE DELIVERY

Temperature:

Pulse:

Respiration:

Fundal height:

Uterus:

Vaginal bleeding:

NURSING PROCESS

List of nursing diagnosis:

NURSING CARE PLAN

Assessment	NSG Diagnosis	Objective	Intervention	Implementation	Evaluation

Assessment	NSG Diagnosis	Objective	Intervention	Implementation	Evaluation

NURSING CARE PLAN

Assessment	NSG Diagnosis	Objective	Intervention	Implementation	Evaluation

Assessment	NSG Diagnosis	Objective	Intervention	Implementation	Evaluation

BIBLIOGRAPHY

PERSONAL HISTORY

Name:

Age:

Date of visit:

Marital status:

Address:

SOCIO ECONOMIC HISTORY

Education of the mother:

Education of her husband:

Occupation:

Income:

Religion:

FAMILY HISTORY

Type of family:

No. of persons in the family:

History of any disease in family:

Family tree:

PREVIOUS MEDICAL AND SURGICAL HISTORY

MENSTRUAL HISTORY

OBSTETRICAL HISTORY

Date	Abortion	Preterm	Fullterm	Type of Delivery	Sex	Alive	Wt	Stillbirth	Remarks

ANTENATAL ATTENDANCE

Date	Wt	Urine Alb. Sugar	BP	FHR	Weeks of Gestation	Fundal Ht	Treatment/Remarks

INVESTIGATION

Blood group:

Hb:

VDRL:

Rh :

ADMISSION TO LABOR ROOM

Admission on:---------------------at---------am/pm.

Contraction commenced on----------------------at-----------am/pm.

Period of gestation:

Membranes: Intact/ruptured on -----------------------at---------am/pm.

Contractions:

Presentation:

Position:

Head engaged/not:

FHR:

Bladder/bowels:

Special observation if, any:

LABOR

Time	BP	Pulse	FHR	Observation	Nursing Care	Intake	Output

DELIVERY RECORD

Membranes ruptured at--------------

Spontaneously/artificially means reason---------------------------

Expulsive contraction commenced at------------------- on------------------

DELIVERY OF BABY

Baby born at---------------------- on------------------------------

Sex:

Apgar Score:

Condition at birth: Active/limp/asphyxiated
Stillborn/macerated means cause----------------------

DELIVERY OF PLACENTA AND MEMBRANES

Delivered at------------------- am/pm.

Spontaneously/helped/manually

Type of placenta: Healthy/infarcts----------- %

Complete/incomplete

Weight:

Cord insertion:

Cord length:

BLOOD LOSS

Before delivery of placenta ----------------------------

During delivery of placenta ----------------------------

After delivery of placenta ----------------------------

Total ----------------------------

PERINEUM

Intact/episiotomy Torn/degree

Type of episiotomy:

Repaired with :

DRUG CHART

S. No.	Name of the Drug	Dose/Route	Action	Indication	Contraindication	Side Effects	Nurses Responsibility

LABOR SUMMARY

Type of labor:

Mode of delivery:

Length of labor:

I stage ---------------hours-------------minutes

II stage ---------------hours-------------minutes

III stage ---------------hours-------------minutes

Total ------------------hours-------------minutes

I Year

PARTOGRAPH

Patient Name ....
Age ....
Ward ....
Gravida ....
Para ....
Obstetrician ....

Date ....

Time							
Pulse rate							
Temperature							

Fetal Heart Rate / MATERNAL BLOOD PRESSURE															
180															
160															
140															
120															
100															
80															
60															
40															

Uterine Contractions in 10 Minutes														
<20 Sec														
20-40 Sec														
>40 Sec														

Vaginal Examinations															
Descend	Dilation														
-5	10														
-4	9														
-3	8														
-2	7														
-1	6														
0	5														
+1	4														
+2	3														
+3	2														
+4	1														
+5	0														

Amniotic fluid														
Presentation														
Position of Vertex/Breech	○	○	○	○	○	○	○	○	○	○	○	○	○	○
Effacement														
Caput														
Moulding														
Oxytocin, Units														
Medication														
I.V. Infusion														
Urine														

CONDITION FOLLOWING THE DELIVERY

Temperature:

Pulse:

Respiration:

Fundal height:

Uterus:

Vaginal bleeding:

NURSING PROCESS

List of nursing diagnosis:

NURSING CARE PLAN

Assessment	NSG Diagnosis	Objective	Intervention	Implementation	Evaluation

Assessment	NSG Diagnosis	Objective	Intervention	Implementation	Evaluation

NURSING CARE PLAN

Assessment	NSG Diagnosis	Objective	Intervention	Implementation	Evaluation

Assessment	NSG Diagnosis	Objective	Intervention	Implementation	Evaluation

BIBLIOGRAPHY

PERSONAL HISTORY

Name:

Age:

Date of visit:

Marital status:

Address:

SOCIOECONOMIC HISTORY

Education of the mother:

Education of her husband:

Occupation:

Income:

Religion:

FAMILY HISTORY

Type of family:

No. of persons in the family:

History of any disease in family:

Family tree:

PREVIOUS MEDICAL AND SURGICAL HISTORY

MENSTRUAL HISTORY

OBSTETRICAL HISTORY

Date	Abortion	Preterm	Fullterm	Type of Delivery	Sex	Alive	Wt	Stillbirth	Remarks

ANTENATAL ATTENDANCE

Date	Wt	Urine Alb. Sugar	BP	FHR	Weeks of Destation	Fundal Ht	Treatment/Remarks

INVESTIGATION

Blood group:

Hb:

VDRL:

Rh:

ADMISSION TO LABOR ROOM

Admission on:--------------------at---------am/pm.

Contraction commenced on----------------------at-----------am/pm.

Period of gestation:

Membranes: Intact/ruptured on -----------------------at--------am/pm.

Contractions:

Presentation:

Position:

Head engaged/not:

FHR:

Bladder/bowels:

Special observation if, any:

LABOR

Time	BP	Pulse	FHR	Observation	Nursing Care	Intake	Output

DELIVERY RECORD

Membranes ruptured at--------------

Spontaneously/artificially means reason-----------------------------

Expulsive contraction commenced at-------------------- on--------------------

DELIVERY OF BABY

Baby born at----------------------- on------------------------------

Sex:

Apgar Score:

Condition at birth: Active/limp/asphyxiated
Stillborn/macerated means cause----------------------

DELIVERY OF PLACENTA AND MEMBRANES

Delivered at------------------- am/pm.

Spontaneously/helped/manually

Type of placenta: Healthy/infarcts----------- %

Complete/incomplete

Weight:

Cord insertion:

Cord length:

BLOOD LOSS

Before delivery of placenta ----------------------------

During delivery of placenta ----------------------------

After delivery of placenta ----------------------------

Total ----------------------------

PERINEUM

Intact/episiotomy Torn/degree

Type of episiotomy:

Repaired with:

DRUG CHART

S. No.	Name of the Drug	Dose/Route	Action	Indication	Contraindication	Side Effects	Nurses Responsibility

LABOR SUMMARY

Type of labor:

Mode of delivery:

Length of labor:

I stage ---------------hours-------------minutes

II stage ---------------hours-------------minutes

III stage ---------------hours-------------minutes

Total ----------------hours-------------minutes

PARTOGRAPH

Patient Name ....
Age ....
Ward ....
Gravida ....
Para ....
Obstetrician ....

Date ....

Time														
Pulse rate														
Temperature														

Fetal Heart Rate / MATERNAL BLOOD PRESSURE														
180														
160														
140														
120														
100														
80														
60														
40														

Uterine Contractions in 10 Minutes (<20 Sec; 20-40 Sec; >40 Sec)														

Vaginal Examinations

Descend	Dilation														
-5	10														
-4	9														
-3	8														
-2	7														
-1	6														
0	5														
+1	4														
+2	3														
+3	2														
+4	1														
+5	0														

Amniotic fluid														
Presentation														
Position of Vertex/Breech	○	○	○	○	○	○	○	○	○	○	○	○	○	○
Effacement														
Caput														
Moulding														
Oxytocin, Units														
Medication														
I.V. Infusion														
Urine														

CONDITION FOLLOWING THE DELIVERY

Temperature:

Pulse:

Respiration:

Fundal height:

Uterus:

Vaginal bleeding:

NURSING PROCESS

List of nursing diagnosis:

NURSING CARE PLAN

Assessment	NSG Diagnosis	Objective	Intervention	Implementation	Evaluation

Assessment	NSG Diagnosis	Objective	Intervention	Implementation	Evaluation

NURSING CARE PLAN

Assessment	NSG Diagnosis	Objective	Intervention	Implementation	Evaluation

Assessment	NSG Diagnosis	Objective	Intervention	Implementation	Evaluation

BIBLIOGRAPHY

POSTNATAL CARE PLAN WITH NURSING THEORY APPLICATION

POSTNATAL CARE PLAN

Name of the hospital/maternity center:

Date of care started:

Date of care ended:

PERSONAL HISTORY

Name:

Age:

Date of visit:

Marital status:

Address:

SOCIOECONOMIC HISTORY

Education of the mother:

Education of her husband:

Occupation:

Income:

Religion:

FAMILY HISTORY

Type of family:

No. of persons in the family:

History of any disease in family:

Family tree:

PREVIOUS MEDICAL AND SURGICAL HISTORY

MENSTRUAL HISTORY

OBSTETRICAL HISTORY

Date	Abortion	Preterm	Fullterm	Type of Delivery	Sex	Alive	Wt	Stillbirth	Remarks

ANTENATAL ATTENDANCE

Date	Wt	Urine		BP	FHR	Weeks of Gestation	Fundal Ht	Treatment/Remarks
		Alb.	Sugar					

INVESTIGATION

Blood group:

Hb:

VDRL:

Rh:

ADMISSION TO LABOR ROOM

Admission on---------------------at----------am/pm.

Contraction commenced on----------------------at------------am/pm.

Period of gestation:

Membranes: Intact/ruptured on -----------------------at---------am/pm.

Contractions:

Presentation:

Position:

Head engaged/not:

FHR:

Bladder/bowels:

Special observation if, any:

LABOR

Time	BP	Pulse	FHR	Observation	Nursing Care	Intake	Output

DELIVERY RECORD

Membranes ruptured at--------------

Spontaneously/artificially means reason----------------------------

Expulsive contraction commenced at-------------------- on--------------------

DELIVERY OF BABY

Baby born at----------------------- on-----------------------------

Sex:

Apgar Score:

Condition at birth: Active/limp/asphyxiated

Stillborn/macerated means cause-----------------------

DELIVERY OF PLACENTA AND MEMBRANES

Delivered at------------------- am/pm.

Spontaneously/helped/manually

Type of placenta: Healthy/infarcts----------- %

Complete/incomplete

Weight:

Cord insertion:

Cord length:

BLOOD LOSS

Before delivery of placenta ---------------

During delivery of placenta ---------------

After delivery of placenta ---------------

Total ---------------

PERINEUM

Intact/episiotomy Torn/degree

Type of episiotomy:

Repaired with:

LABOR SUMMARY

Type of labor:

Mode of delivery:

Length of labor:

I stage --------------hours------------minutes

II stage ---------------hours------------minutes

III stage --------------hours------------minutes

Total ---------------hours------------minutes

CONDITION FOLLOWING THE DELIVERY

Temperature:

Pulse:

Respiration:

Fundal height:

Uterus:

Vaginal bleeding:

DRUG CHART

S. No.	Name of the Drug	Dose/Route	Action	Indication	Contraindication	Side Effects	Nurses Responsibility

CLINICAL CHART OF PUERPERIUM

Date															Fundal height
	M	E	M	E	M	E	M	E	M	E	M	E	M	E	
Temperature															
Pulse															
Respiration															
BP															
Lochia															
Urine															
Motion															

CLINICAL CHART OF BABY

Date														
	M	E	M	E	M	E	M	E	M	E	M	E	M	E
Temperature														
Pulse														
Respiration														
BP														
Weight														
Urine														
Motion														

NURSING PROCESS

List of nursing diagnosis:

NURSING CARE PLAN

Assessment	NSG Diagnosis	Objective	Intervention	Implementation	Evaluation

NURSING CARE PLAN

Assessment	NSG Diagnosis	Objective	Intervention	Implementation	Evaluation

NURSING CARE PLAN

Assessment	NSG Diagnosis	Objective	Intervention	Implementation	Evaluation

NURSING CARE PLAN

Assessment	NSG Diagnosis	Objective	Intervention	Implementation	Evaluation

DISCHARGE SUMMARY/HEALTH EDUCATION

POSTNATAL CARE PLAN

Name of the hospital/maternity center:

Date of care started:

Date of care ended:

PERSONAL HISTORY

Name:

Age:

Date of visit:

Marital status:

Address:

SOCIOECONOMIC HISTORY

Education of the mother:

Education of her husband:

Occupation:

Income:

Religion:

FAMILY HISTORY

Type of family:

No. of persons in the family:

History of any disease in family:

Family tree:

PREVIOUS MEDICAL AND SURGICAL HISTORY

MENSTRUAL HISTORY

OBSTETRICAL HISTORY

Date	Abortion	Preterm	Fullterm	Type of Delivery	Sex	Alive	Wt	Stillbirth	Remarks

ANTENATAL ATTENDANCE

Date	Wt	Urine		BP	FHR	Weeks of Gestation	Fundal Ht	Treatment/Remarks
		Alb.	Sugar					

INVESTIGATION

Blood group:

Hb:

VDRL:

Rh:

ADMISSION TO LABOR ROOM

Admission on:---------------------at---------am/pm.

Contraction commenced on----------------------at-----------am/pm.

Period of gestation:

Membranes: Intact/ruptured on ------------------------at--------am/pm.

Contractions:

Presentation:

Position:

Head engaged/not:

FHR:

Bladder/bowels:

Special observation if, any:

LABOR

Time	BP	Pulse	FHR	Observation	Nursing Care	Intake	Output

DELIVERY RECORD

Membranes ruptured at--------------

Spontaneously/artificially means reason----------------------------

Expulsive contraction commenced at-------------------- on--------------------

DELIVERY OF BABY

Baby born at----------------------- on-----------------------------

Sex:

Apgar Score:

Condition at birth: Active/limp/asphyxiated
Stillborn/macerated means cause----------------------

DELIVERY OF PLACENTA AND MEMBRANES

Delivered at------------------- am/pm.

Spontaneously/helped/manually

Type of placenta: Healthy/infarcts----------- %

Complete/incomplete

Weight:

Cord insertion:

Cord length:

BLOOD LOSS

Before delivery of placenta ----------------

During delivery of placenta ----------------

After delivery of placenta ----------------

Total ----------------

PERINEUM

Intact/episiotomy Torn/degree

Type of episiotomy:

Repaired with:

DRUG CHART

S. No.	Name of the Drug	Dose/Route	Action	Indication	Contraindication	Side Effects	Nurses Responsibility

LABOR SUMMARY

Type of labor:

Mode of delivery:

Length of labor:

I stage --------------hours-------------minutes

II stage --------------hours-------------minutes

III stage --------------hours-------------minutes

Total --------------hours-------------minutes

CONDITION FOLLOWING THE DELIVERY

Temperature:

Pulse:

Respiration:

Fundal height:

Uterus:

Vaginal bleeding:

CLINICAL CHART OF PUERPERIUM

Date															Fundal height
	M	E	M	E	M	E	M	E	M	E	M	E	M	E	
Temperature															
Pulse															
Respiration															
BP															
Lochia															
Urine															
Motion															

CLINICAL CHART OF BABY

Date														
	M	E	M	E	M	E	M	E	M	E	M	E	M	E
Temperature														
Pulse														
Respiration														
BP														
Weight														
Urine														
Motion														

NURSING PROCESS

List of nursing diagnosis:

I Year

NURSING CARE PLAN

Assessment	NSG Diagnosis	Objective	Intervention	Implementation	Evaluation

Assessment	NSG Diagnosis	Objective	Intervention	Implementation	Evaluation

NURSING CARE PLAN

Assessment	NSG Diagnosis	Objective	Intervention	Implementation	Evaluation

Assessment	NSG Diagnosis	Objective	Intervention	Implementation	Evaluation

DISCHARGE SUMMARY/HEALTH EDUCATION

POSTNATAL CARE PLAN

Name of the hospital/maternity center:

Date of care started:

Date of care ended:

PERSONAL HISTORY

Name:

Age:

Date of visit:

Marital status:

Address:

SOCIOECONOMIC HISTORY

Education of the mother:

Education of her husband:

Occupation:

Income:

Religion:

FAMILY HISTORY

Type of family:

No. of persons in the family:

History of any disease in family:

Family tree:

PREVIOUS MEDICAL AND SURGICAL HISTORY

MENSTRUAL HISTORY

OBSTETRICAL HISTORY

Date	Abortion	Preterm	Fullterm	Type of Delivery	Sex	Alive	Wt	Stillbirth	Remarks

ANTENATAL ATTENDANCE

Date	Wt	Urine		BP	FHR	Weeks of Gestation	Fundal Ht	Treatment/Remarks
		Alb.	Sugar					

I Year

INVESTIGATION

Blood group:

Hb:

VDRL:

Rh:

ADMISSION TO LABOR ROOM

Admission on:--------------------at---------am/pm.

Contraction commenced on----------------------at-----------am/pm.

Period of gestation:

Membranes: Intact/ruptured on -----------------------at--------am/pm.

Contractions:

Presentation:

Position:

Head engaged/not:

FHR:

Bladder/bowels:

Special observation if, any:

LABOR

Time	BP	Pulse	FHR	Observation	Nursing Care	Intake	Output

DELIVERY RECORD

Membranes ruptured at--------------

Spontaneously/artificially means reason----------------------------

Expulsive contraction commenced at-------------------- on--------------------

DELIVERY OF BABY

Baby born at----------------------- on------------------------------

Sex:

Apgar Score:

Condition at birth: Active/limp/asphyxiated
Stillborn/macerated means cause----------------------

DELIVERY OF PLACENTA AND MEMBRANES

Delivered at-------------------- am/pm.

Spontaneously/helped/manually

Type of placenta: Healthy/infarcts----------- %

Complete/incomplete

Weight:

Cord insertion:

Cord length:

BLOOD LOSS

Before delivery of placenta ----------------

During delivery of placenta ----------------

After delivery of placenta ----------------

Total ----------------

PERINEUM

Intact/episiotomy Torn/degree

Type of episiotomy:

Repaired with:

DRUG CHART

S. No.	Name of the Drug	Dose/Route	Action	Indication	Contraindication	Side Effects	Nurses Responsibility

LABOR SUMMARY

Type of labor:

Mode of delivery:

Length of labor:

I stage --------------hours-------------minutes

II stage --------------hours-------------minutes

III stage --------------hours-------------minutes

Total ---------------hours-------------minutes

CONDITION FOLLOWING THE DELIVERY

Temperature:

Pulse:

Respiration:

Fundal height:

Uterus:

Vaginal bleeding:

CLINICAL CHART OF PUERPERIUM

Date															Fundal height
	M	E	M	E	M	E	M	E	M	E	M	E	M	E	
Temperature															
Pulse															
Respiration															
BP															
Lochia															
Urine															
Motion															

CLINICAL CHART OF BABY

Date														
	M	E	M	E	M	E	M	E	M	E	M	E	M	E
Temperature														
Pulse														
Respiration														
BP														
Weight														
Urine														
Motion														

NURSING PROCESS

List of nursing diagnosis:

NURSING CARE PLAN

Assessment	NSG Diagnosis	Objective	Intervention	Implementation	Evaluation

Assessment	NSG Diagnosis	Objective	Intervention	Implementation	Evaluation

NURSING CARE PLAN

Assessment	NSG Diagnosis	Objective	Intervention	Implementation	Evaluation

Assessment	NSG Diagnosis	Objective	Intervention	Implementation	Evaluation

DISCHARGE SUMMARY/HEALTH EDUCATION

BIBLIOGRAPHY

NEWBORN CARE PLAN WITH THEORY APPLICATION

NEWBORN CARE PLAN

Name of the baby:

Sex:

Name of the hospital/maternity center:

Date of care started:

Date of care ended:

MOTHERS OBSTETRIC HISTORY

Date	Abortion	Preterm	Fullterm	Type of Delivery	Sex	Alive	Wt	Stillbirth	Remarks

PRESENT PREGNANCY HISTORY

Antenatal History

Antenatal care: Yes/no

Any special observation:

Labor

Type of labor:

Mode of delivery:

Length of labor:

Membranes ruptured: Spontaneously/artificially means reason----------------

Placenta and membranes: Healthy/unhealthy

Cord: length-------------, insertion-----------------

Fetal distress: Present/not

If any other specify---

Drugs given during delivery:

Baby

Date of birth: ---------------------at-----------------am/pm.

Condition at birth:

Apgar Score:

Treatment at birth:

Drugs given:

Feeding: Mother/formula/tube

Baby transferred to --

PHYSICAL EXAMINATION

a. General Condition

b. Weight:

c. Length:

d. Head circumference:

e. Chest circumference:

f. Head to foot examination:

Moulding: Normal/excessive/nil

Caput: Yes/no

Eyes:

Mouth:

Heart:

Lungs:

Abdomen:

Back:

Limbs:

Genitalia:

Rectum:

ANY OTHER FINDINGS

INVESTIGATION

Blood group:

If any other investigation done means specify:

DRUG CHART

S. No.	Name of the Drug	Dose/Route	Action	Indication	Contraindication	Side Effects	Nurses Responsibility

CLINICAL CHART OF BABY

Date														
	M	E	M	E	M	E	M	E	M	E	M	E	M	E
Temperature														
Pulse														
Respiration														
BP														
Weight														
Urine														
Motion														

NURSING PROCESS

List of nursing diagnosis:

THEORY APPLICATION

NURSING CARE PLAN

Assessment	NSG Diagnosis	Objective	Intervention	Implementation	Evaluation

Assessment	NSG Diagnosis	Objective	Intervention	Implementation	Evaluation

NURSING CARE PLAN

Assessment	NSG Diagnosis	Objective	Intervention	Implementation	Evaluation

Assessment	NSG Diagnosis	Objective	Intervention	Implementation	Evaluation

DISCHARGE SUMMARY/HEALTH EDUCATION

BIBLIOGRAPHY

NEWBORN CARE PLAN

Name of the baby:

Sex:

Name of the hospital/maternity center:

Date of care started:

Date of care ended:

MOTHERS OBSTETRIC HISTORY

Date	Abortion	Preterm	Fullterm	Type of Delivery	Sex	Alive	Wt	Stillbirth	Remarks

PRESENT PREGNANCY HISTORY

Antenatal History

Antenatal care: Yes/no

Any special observation:

Labor

Type of labor:

Mode of delivery:

Length of labor:

Membranes ruptured: Spontaneously/artificially means reason----------------

Placenta and membranes: Healthy/unhealthy

Cord: Length-------------, insertion----------------

Fetal distress: Present/not

If any other specify---

Drugs given during delivery:

Baby

Date of birth: ---------------------at-----------------am/pm.

Condition at birth:

Apgar Score:

Treatment at birth:

Drugs given:

Feeding: Mother/formula/tube

Baby transferred to ---------------------------------------

PHYSICAL EXAMINATION

a. General Condition

b. Weight:

c. Length:

d. Head circumference:

e. Chest circumference:

f. Head to foot examination

Moulding: Normal/excessive/nil

Caput: Yes/no

Eyes:

Mouth:

Heart:

Lungs:

Abdomen:

Back:

Limbs:

Genitalia:

Rectum:

ANY OTHER FINDINGS

INVESTIGATION

Blood group:

If any other investigation done means specify:

DRUG CHART

S. No.	Name of the Drug	Dose/Route	Action	Indication	Contraindication	Side Effects	Nurses Responsibility

CLINICAL CHART OF BABY

Date														
	M	E	M	E	M	E	M	E	M	E	M	E	M	E
Temperature														
Pulse														
Respiration														
BP														
Weight														
Urine														
Motion														

NURSING PROCESS

List of nursing diagnosis:

NURSING CARE PLAN

Assessment	NSG Diagnosis	Objective	Intervention	Implementation	Evaluation

Assessment	NSG Diagnosis	Objective	Intervention	Implementation	Evaluation

NURSING CARE PLAN

Assessment	NSG Diagnosis	Objective	Intervention	Implementation	Evaluation

Assessment	NSG Diagnosis	Objective	Intervention	Implementation	Evaluation

DISCHARGE SUMMARY/HEALTH EDUCATION

BIBLIOGRAPHY

GYNECOLOGY CARE PLAN WITH NURSING THEORY APPLICATION

GYNECOLOGY CARE PLAN

PERSONAL DATA

Name:

Age:

Social status:

Chief complaint:

MENSTRUAL HISTORY

Age of onset:

Regularity:

Duration:

Length:

Amount of bleeding:

LMP:

OBSTETRICAL HISTORY

Date	Abortion	Preterm	Fullterm	Type of Delivery	Sex	Alive	Wt	Stillbirth	Remarks

PAST MEDICAL AND SURGICAL HISTORY

Specify any medical gynecological history like

Systemic disorders: Yes/no

Metabolic disorders: Yes/no

Endocrinal disorders: Yes/no

Specify any surgical gynecological history like

Nature of operation:

Anesthetic complication:

Postoperative convalescence:

Histopathological report:

FAMILY HISTORY

If any of the family member has—

Malignancy in the breast, colon ovary, or other genital organs: Yes/no

MARITAL HISTORY

Marital status:

Sexual status: Fertile/infertile

Specify if any contraceptive devices use:

HISTORY OF TAKING ANY MEDICATION

Name of the drug/dosage:

For what purpose:

Duration of taking:

Any allergic medication:

EXAMINATION

General and Systemic

Built: Obese/thin

Nutrition: Average/poor

Stature: Include secondary sexual characters

Color: Pale/jaundice/normal

Teeth, gums, tonsils any septic foci: Yes/no

Neck:

Palpation of thyroid gland:

Palpation of lymph nodes [specially left supraclavicular glands]:

In legs edema present: Yes/no

CVS:

Respiratory system:

Vital signs:

Temperature:

Pulse:

Respiration:

BP:

Gynecological Examination

Breast Examination:

Specify if any abnormality:

Abdominal Examination

Skin condition of the abdomen

Presence of old scar: Yes/no

Presence of striae: Yes/no

Presence of prominent veins: Yes/no

Incisional hernia: Yes/no

Intestinal obstruction: Yes/no

Pelvic peritonitis: Yes/no

Ascites: Yes/no

Pelvic tumors: Yes/no

Pelvic Examination

By observation

Any abnormalities in pubic hair,

Clitoris, labia, perineum: Yes/no

Any vaginal discharge: Yes/no

Any stress incontinence: Yes/no

Any genital prolapse: Yes/no

Any hemorrhoids, anal fissure, anal fistula: Yes/no

Any problem in vaginal cervix:

DRUG CHART

S. No.	Name of the Drug	Dose/Route	Action	Indication	Contraindication	Side Effects	Nurses Responsibility

SPECIAL INVESTIGATION

NURSING PROCESS

List of nursing diagnosis:

NURSING CARE PLAN

Assessment	NSG Diagnosis	Objective	Intervention	Implementation	Evaluation

Assessment	NSG Diagnosis	Objective	Intervention	Implementation	Evaluation

NURSING CARE PLAN

Assessment	NSG Diagnosis	Objective	Intervention	Implementation	Evaluation

Assessment	NSG Diagnosis	Objective	Intervention	Implementation	Evaluation

THEORY APPLICATION

DISCHARGE SUMMARY/HEALTH EDUCATION

BIBLIOGRAPHY

FAMILY PLANNING CARE PLAN WITH NURSING THEORY APPLICATION

FAMILY PLANNING CARE PLAN

Name of the hospital/maternity center:

Date of care started:

Date of care ended:

PERSONAL HISTORY

Name:

Age:

Date of visit:

Marital status:

Address:

SOCIOECONOMIC HISTORY

Education of the mother:

Education of her husband:

Occupation:

Income:

Religion:

FAMILY HISTORY

Type of family:

No. of persons in the family:

History of any disease in family:

Family tree:

PREVIOUS MEDICAL AND SURGICAL HISTORY

MENSTRUAL HISTORY

OBSTETRICAL HISTORY

Date	Abortion	Preterm	Fullterm	Type of Delivery	Sex	Alive	Wt	Stillbirth	Remarks

EXAMINATION

Physical Examination

I Year

Vaginal Examination

Shape of the uterus:

Size of the uterus:

Position of the uterus:

FAMILY PLANNING HISTORY

Previously used any family planning method: Yes/no

Type of family planning: Temporarily/permanent

Drawback of previous method:

PRESENT METHOD AND PROCEDURE OF FAMILY PLANNING

SPECIAL INSTRUCTION TO THE WOMAN

MEDICATION

NURSING PROCESS

List of nursing diagnosis:

NURSING CARE PLAN

Assessment	NSG Diagnosis	Objective	Intervention	Implementation	Evaluation

Assessment	NSG Diagnosis	Objective	Intervention	Implementation	Evaluation

NURSING CARE PLAN

Assessment	NSG Diagnosis	Objective	Intervention	Implementation	Evaluation

Assessment	NSG Diagnosis	Objective	Intervention	Implementation	Evaluation

DISCHARGE SUMMARY/HEALTH EDUCATION

BIBLIOGRAPHY

ANTENATAL CASE STUDY

INTRODUCTION

HISTORY COLLECTION

Name of the hospital/maternity center:

Date of care started:

Date of care ended:

Personal History

Name:

Age:

Date of visit:

Marital status:

Address:

Socioeconomic History

Education of the mother:

Education of her husband:

Occupation:

Income:

Religion:

Family History

Type of family:

No. of persons in the family:

History of any disease in family:

Family tree:

Previous Medical and Surgical History

Menstrual History

Obstetrical History

Date	Abortion	Preterm	Fullterm	Type of Delivery	Sex	Alive	Wt	Stillbirth	Remarks

Antenatal Attendance

Date	Wt	Urine		BP	FHR	Weeks of Gestation	Fundal Ht	Treatment/Remarks
		Alb.	Sugar					

INVESTIGATION

Blood group:

Hb:

VDRL:

Rh:

PHYSICAL EXAMINATION

a. General Condition:

Heart:

Lungs:

Mouth:

Breast and nipples:

Abdomen:

Perineum:

Legs and feet:

Any others if, specify:

b. Symptoms

Pain:

Appetite:

Heart burn:

Micturition:

DRUG CHART

S. No.	Name of the Drug	Dose/Route	Action	Indication	Contraindication	Side Effects	Nurses Responsibility

Vaginal discharge:

Other:

C. Obstetrical Examination

Period of gestation:

Presentation:

Position:

Height of fundus:

Head: Engaged/not

Fetal heart rate:

NURSING MANAGEMENT

List of nursing diagnosis:

NURSING CARE PLAN

Assessment	NSG Diagnosis	Objective	Intervention	Implementation	Evaluation

Assessment	NSG Diagnosis	Objective	Intervention	Implementation	Evaluation

NURSING CARE PLAN

Assessment	NSG Diagnosis	Objective	Intervention	Implementation	Evaluation

Assessment	NSG Diagnosis	Objective	Intervention	Implementation	Evaluation

NURSING CARE PLAN

Assessment	NSG Diagnosis	Objective	Intervention	Implementation	Evaluation

Assessment	NSG Diagnosis	Objective	Intervention	Implementation	Evaluation

PROGRESS NOTES

Date	Nursing Care Given

CONCLUSION

BIBLIOGRAPHY

NATAL CASE STUDY

INTRODUCTION

HISTORY COLLECTION

Name of the hospital/maternity center:

Date of care started:

Date of care ended:

Personal History

Name:

Age:

Date of visit:

Marital status:

Address:

Socioeconomic History

Education of the mother:

Education of her husband:

Occupation:

Income:

Religion:

Family History

Type of family:

No. of persons in the family:

History of any disease in family:

Family tree:

Previous Medical and Surgical History

Menstrual History

Obstetrical History

Date	Abortion	Preterm	Fullterm	Type of Delivery	Sex	Alive	Wt	Stillbirth	Remarks

Antenatal Attendance

Date	Wt	Urine		BP	FHR	Weeks of Gestation	Fundal Ht	Treatment/Remarks
		Alb.	Sugar					

INVESTIGATION

Blood group:

Hb:

VDRL:

Rh:

ANATOMY AND PHYSIOLOGY OF NATAL

PARTOGRAPH

Patient Name ....
Age ....
Ward ....
Gravida ....
Para ....
Obstetrician ....

Date ....

Time														
Pulse rate														
Temperature														

Fetal Heart Rate / MATERNAL / BLOOD PRESSURE																													
	180																												
	160																												
	140																												
	120																												
	100																												
	80																												
	60																												
	40																												

Uterine Contractions in 10 Minutes <20 Sec 20-40 Sec >40 Sec														

Vaginal Examinations															
Descend	Dilation														
-5	10														
-4	9														
-3	8														
-2	7														
-1	6														
0	5														
+1	4														
+2	3														
+3	2														
+4	1														
+5	0														

Amniotic fluid														
Presentation														
Position of Vertex/Breech														
Effacement														
Caput														
Moulding														
Oxytocin, Units														
Medication														
I.V. Infusion														
Urine														

ADMISSION TO LABOR ROOM

Admission on:---------------------at----------am/pm.

Contraction commenced on----------------------at-----------am/pm.

Period of gestation:

Membranes: Intact/ruptured on -----------------------at--------am/pm.

Contractions:

Presentation:

Position:

Head engaged/not:

FHR:

Bladder/bowels:

Special observation if, any:

DELIVERY RECORD

Membranes ruptured at--------------

Spontaneously/artificially means reason---------------------------

Expulsive contraction commenced at------------------- on-------------------

DELIVERY OF BABY

Baby born at---------------------- on-----------------------------

Sex:

Apgar Score:

Condition at birth: Active/limp/asphyxiated

Stillborn/macerated means cause----------------------

DELIVERY OF PLACENTA AND MEMBRANES

Delivered at------------------ am/pm.

Spontaneously/helped/manually

Type of placenta: Healthy/infarcts----------- %

Complete/incomplete

Weight:

Cord insertion:

Cord length:

BLOOD LOSS

Before delivery of placenta ----------------

During delivery of placenta ----------------

After delivery of placenta ----------------

Total ----------------

PERINEUM

Intact/episiotomy Torn/degree

Type of episiotomy:

Repaired with:

LABOR SUMMARY

Type of labor:

Mode of delivery:

Length of labor:

I stage ---------------hours------------minutes

II stage ---------------hours------------minutes

III stage ---------------hours------------minutes

Total ----------------hours-------------minutes

CONDITION FOLLOWING THE DELIVERY

Temperature:

Pulse:

Respiration:

Fundal height:

Uterus:

Vaginal bleeding:

DRUG CHART

S. No.	Name of the Drug	Dose/Route	Action	Indication	Contraindication	Side Effects	Nurses Responsibility

NURSING MANAGEMENT

List of nursing diagnosis:

THEORY APPLICATION

PROGRESS NOTES

NURSING CARE PLAN

Assessment	NSG Diagnosis	Objective	Intervention	Implementation	Evaluation

Assessment	NSG Diagnosis	Objective	Intervention	Implementation	Evaluation

NURSING CARE PLAN

Assessment	NSG Diagnosis	Objective	Intervention	Implementation	Evaluation

Assessment	NSG Diagnosis	Objective	Intervention	Implementation	Evaluation

NURSING CARE PLAN

Assessment	NSG Diagnosis	Objective	Intervention	Implementation	Evaluation

Assessment	NSG Diagnosis	Objective	Intervention	Implementation	Evaluation

BIBLIOGRAPHY

POSTNATAL CASE STUDY

HISTORY COLLECTION

Name of the hospital/maternity center:

Date of care started:

Date of care ended:

Personal History

Name:

Age:

Date of visit:

Marital status:

Address:

Socioeconomic History

Education of the mother:

Education of her husband:

Occupation:

Income:

Religion:

Family History

Type of family:

No. of persons in the family:

History of any disease in family:

Family tree:

Previous Medical and Surgical History

Menstrual History

Obstetrical History

Date	Abortion	Preterm	Fullterm	Type of Delivery	Sex	Alive	Wt	Stillbirth	Remarks

Antenatal Attendance

Date	Wt	Urine		BP	FHR	Weeks of Gestation	Fundal Ht	Treatment/Remarks
		Alb.	Sugar					

INVESTIGATION

Blood group:

Hb:

VDRL:

Rh:

ANATOMY AND PHYSIOLOGY OF POSTNATAL

ADMISSION TO LABOR ROOM

Admission on:--------------------at----------am/pm.

Contraction commenced on----------------------at-----------am/pm.

Period of gestation:

Membranes: Intact/ruptured on -----------------------at---------am/pm.

Contractions:

Presentation:

Position:

Head engaged/not:

FHR:

Bladder/bowels:

Special observation if, any:

PARTOGRAM

PARTOGRAPH

Patient Name ....
Age ....
Ward ....
Gravida ....
Para ....
Obstetrician ....

Date ....

Time														
Pulse rate														
Temperature														

Fetal Heart Rate / MATERNAL BLOOD PRESSURE																												
180																												
160																												
140																												
120																												
100																												
80																												
60																												
40																												

Uterine Contractions in 10 Minutes (<20 Sec; 20-40 Sec; >40 Sec)														

Vaginal Examinations

Descend	Dilation														
-5	10														
-4	9														
-3	8														
-2	7														
-1	6														
0	5														
+1	4														
+2	3														
+3	2														
+4	1														
+5	0														

Amniotic fluid														
Presentation														
Position of Vertex/Breech	○	○	○	○	○	○	○	○	○	○	○	○	○	○
Effacement														
Caput														
Moulding														
Oxytocin, Units														
Medication														
I.V. Infusion														
Urine														

DELIVERY RECORD

Membranes ruptured at---------------,

Spontaneously/artificially means reason------------------------------

Expulsive contraction commenced at--------------------- on--------------------

DELIVERY OF BABY

Baby born at----------------------- on------------------------------

Sex:

Apgar Score:

Condition at birth: Active/limp/asphyxiated

Stillborn/macerated means cause-----------------------

DELIVERY OF PLACENTA AND MEMBRANES

Delivered at------------------- am/pm.

Spontaneously/helped/manually

Type of placenta: Healthy/infarcts----------- %

Complete/incomplete

Weight:

Cord insertion:

Cord length:

BLOOD LOSS

Before delivery of placenta ----------------

During delivery of placenta ----------------

After delivery of placenta ----------------

Total ----------------

PERINEUM

Intact/episiotomy Torn/degree

Type of episiotomy:

Repaired with:

LABOR SUMMARY

Type of labor:

Mode of delivery:

Length of labor:

I stage --------------hours-------------minutes

II stage -------------hours--------------minutes

III stage -------------hours--------------minutes

Total --------------hours--------------minutes

CONDITION FOLLOWING THE DELIVERY

Temperature:

Pulse:

Respiration:

Fundal height:

Uterus:

Vaginal bleeding:

DRUG CHART

S. No.	Name of the Drug	Dose/Route	Action	Indication	Contraindication	Side Effects	Nurses Responsibility

CLINICAL CHART OF BABY

Date														
	M	E	M	E	M	E	M	E	M	E	M	E	M	E
Temperature														
Pulse														
Respiration														
BP														
Weight														
Urine														
Motion														

CLINICAL CHART OF PUERPERIUM

Date															Fundal height
	M	E	M	E	M	E	M	E	M	E	M	E	M	E	
Temperature															
Pulse															
Respiration															
BP															
Lochia															
Urine															
Motion															

NURSING MANAGEMENT

List of nursing diagnosis:

PROGRESS NOTES

Date	Nursing Care Given

THEORY APPLICATION

DISCHARGE SUMMARY/HEALTH EDUCATION

NURSING CARE PLAN

Assessment	NSG Diagnosis	Objective	Intervention	Implementation	Evaluation

Assessment	NSG Diagnosis	Objective	Intervention	Implementation	Evaluation

NURSING CARE PLAN

Assessment	NSG Diagnosis	Objective	Intervention	Implementation	Evaluation

Assessment	NSG Diagnosis	Objective	Intervention	Implementation	Evaluation

NURSING CARE PLAN

Assessment	NSG Diagnosis	Objective	Intervention	Implementation	Evaluation

Assessment	NSG Diagnosis	Objective	Intervention	Implementation	Evaluation

NEWBORN CASE STUDY

INTRODUCTION

HISTORY

Name of the baby:

Sex:

Name of the hospital/ maternity center:

Date of care started:

Date of care ended:

Mothers Obstetric History

Date	Abortion	Preterm	Fullterm	Type of Delivery	Sex	Alive	Wt	Stillbirth	Remarks

Present Pregnancy History

A. Antenatal History

Antenatal care: Yes/no

Any special observation:

B. Labor

Type of labor:

Mode of delivery:

Length of labor:

Membranes ruptured: Spontaneously/artificially means reason----------------

Placenta and membranes: Healthy/unhealthy

Cord: Length------------, insertion-----------------

Fetal distress: Present/not

If any other specify:

Drugs given during delivery:

C. Baby

Date of birth: ---------------------at-----------------am/pm.

Condition at birth:

Apgar Score:

Treatment at birth:

Drugs given:

Feeding: Mother/formula/tube

Baby transferred to --

PHYSICAL EXAMINATION

a. General condition:

b. Weight:

c. Length:

d. Head circumference:

e. Chest circumference:

f. Head to foot examination

Moulding: Normal/excessive/nil

Caput: Yes/no

Eyes:

Mouth:

Heart:

Lungs:

Abdomen:

Back:

Limbs:

Genitalia:

Rectum:

Any other findings:

INVESTIGATION

Blood group:

If any other investigation done means specify:

DRUG CHART

S. No.	Name of the Drug	Dose/Route	Action	Indication	Contraindication	Side Effects	Nurses Responsibility

ANATOMY PHYSIOLOGY RELATED TO NEWBORN

NURSING MANAGEMENT

List of nursing diagnosis:

I Year

NURSING CARE PLAN

Assessment	NSG Diagnosis	Objective	Intervention	Implementation	Evaluation

Assessment	NSG Diagnosis	Objective	Intervention	Implementation	Evaluation

NURSING CARE PLAN

Assessment	NSG Diagnosis	Objective	Intervention	Implementation	Evaluation

Assessment	NSG Diagnosis	Objective	Intervention	Implementation	Evaluation

NURSING CARE PLAN

Assessment	NSG Diagnosis	Objective	Intervention	Implementation	Evaluation

Assessment	NSG Diagnosis	Objective	Intervention	Implementation	Evaluation

PROGRESS NOTES

Clinical Chart of Baby

Date														
	M	E	M	E	M	E	M	E	M	E	M	E	M	E
Temperature														
Pulse														
Respiration														
BP														
Weight														
Urine														
Motion														

DISCHARGE SUMMARY/HEALTH EDUCATION

BIBLIOGRAPHY

GYNECOLOGY CASE STUDY

INTRODUCTION

HISTORY

Personal Data

Name:

Age:

Social status:

Chief complaint:

Menstrual History

Age of onset:

Regularity:

Duration:

Length:

Amount of bleeding:

LMP:

Obstetrical History

Date	Abortion	Preterm	Fullterm	Type of Delivery	Sex	Alive	Wt	Stillbirth	Remarks

I Year

Past Medical and Surgical History

- Specify any medical gynecological history like

  Systemic disorders: Yes/no

  Metabolic disorders: Yes/no

  Endocrinal disorders: Yes/no

- Specify any surgical gynecological history like

  Nature of operation:

  Anesthetic complication:

  Postoperative convalescence:

  Histopathological report:

Family History

If any of the family member has—

Malignancy in the breast, colon, ovary, or other genital organs: Yes/no

Marital History

Marital status:

Sexual status: Fertile/infertile

Specify If any contraceptive devices use:

History of Taking any Medication

Name of the drug/dosage:

For what purpose:

Duration of taking:

Any allergic medication:

EXAMINATION

General and Systemic

Built: Obese/thin

Nutrition: Average/poor

Stature: [include secondary sexual characters]

Color: Pale/jaundice/normal

Teeth, gums, tonsils any septic foci: Yes/no

Neck:

Palpation of thyroid gland:

Palpation of lymph nodes [specially left supraclavicular glands]:

In legs edema present: Yes/no

CVS:

Respiratory system:

Vital Signs:

Temperature:

Pulse:

Respiration:

BP:

Gynecological Examination

1. Breast examination:

    Specify if any abnormality:

2. Abdominal examination

    Skin condition of the abdomen

    Presence of old scar: Yes/no

    Presence of striae: Yes/no

    Presence of prominent veins: Yes/no

    Incisional hernia: Yes/no

    Intestinal obstruction: Yes/no

    Pelvic peritonitis: Yes/no

    Ascites: Yes/no

    Pelvic tumors: Yes/no

3. Pelvic examination

    By observation

    Any abnormalities in pubic hair,

clitoris, labia, perineum: Yes/no

Any vaginal discharge: Yes/no

Any stress incontinence: Yes/no

Any genital prolapsed: Yes/no

Any hemorrhoids, anal fissure, anal fistula: Yes/no

Any problem in vaginal cervix:

SPECIAL INVESTIGATION

DRUG CHART

S. No.	Name of the Drug	Dose/Route	Action	Indication	Contraindication	Side Effects	Nurses Responsibility

NURSING MANAGEMENT

List of nursing diagnosis:

NURSING CARE PLAN

Assessment	NSG Diagnosis	Objective	Intervention	Implementation	Evaluation

Assessment	NSG Diagnosis	Objective	Intervention	Implementation	Evaluation

NURSING CARE PLAN

Assessment	NSG Diagnosis	Objective	Intervention	Implementation	Evaluation

Assessment	NSG Diagnosis	Objective	Intervention	Implementation	Evaluation

NURSING CARE PLAN

Assessment	NSG Diagnosis	Objective	Intervention	Implementation	Evaluation

Assessment	NSG Diagnosis	Objective	Intervention	Implementation	Evaluation

PROGRESS NOTES

Date	Nursing Care Given

DISCHARGE SUMMARY AND HEALTH EDUCATION

BIBLIOGRAPHY

PARTOGRAPH

Patient Name ....
Age ....
Ward ....
Gravida ....
Para ....
Obstetrician ....

Date ....

Time														
Pulse rate														
Temperature														

Fetal Heart Rate	MATERNAL	BLOOD PRESSURE																													
			180																												
			160																												
			140																												
			120																												
			100																												
			80																												
			60																												
			40																												

Uterine Contractions in 10 Minutes <20 Sec 20-40 Sec >40 Sec														

Vaginal Examinations															
Descend	Dilation														
-5	10														
-4	9														
-3	8														
-2	7														
-1	6														
0	5														
+1	4														
+2	3														
+3	2														
+4	1														
+5	0														

Amniotic fluid														
Presentation														
Position of Vertex/Breech	○	○	○	○	○	○	○	○	○	○	○	○	○	○
Effacement														
Caput														
Moulding														
Oxytocin, Units														
Medication														
I.V. Infusion														
Urine														

CLINICAL SPECIALTY-I
OBSTETRIC AND GYNECOLOGICAL NURSING

Placement: 1st year

Hours of Instruction
Theory: 150 Hours
Practical: 650 Hours
Total: 800 Hours

Course Description

This course is designed to assist students in developming expertise and in-depth understanding in the field of obstetric and gynecological nursing. It will help students to appreciate the client as a holistic individual and develop skill to function as an independent midwifery practitioner. It will further enable the student to function as educator, manager, and researcher in the field of obstetric and gynecological nursing.

Objectives

At the end of the course the students will be able to:

1. Appreciate the trends in the field of midwifery, obstetrics and gynecology as a specialty.
2. Describe the population dynamics and indicators of maternal and child health.
3. Describe the concepts of biophysical, psychological and spiritual aspects of normal pregnancy, labor and puerperium.
4. Provide comprehensive nursing care to women during reproductive period and newborns.
5. Integrate the concepts of family centered nursing care and nursing process approach in obstetric and gynecological nursing.
6. Identify and analyze the deviations from normal birth process and refer appropriately.
7. Describe the pharmacological agents, their effects during pregnancy, child birth, puerperium, lactation and the role of nurse.
8. Counsel adolescents, women and families on issues pertaining to pregnancy, child birth and lactation
9. describe the role of various types of complementary and alternative therapies in obstetric and gynecological nursing.
10. Incorporate evidence based nursing practice and identify the areas of research in the field of obstetric and gynaecological nursing.
11. Describe the recent advancement in contraceptive technology and birth control measures.
12. Appreciate the legal and ethical issues pertaining to obstetric and gynecological nursing.

Course Content

Units	Hours	Content
I	10	**Introduction** ❑ Historical and contemporary perspectives ❑ Epidemiological aspects of maternal and child birth ❑ Magnitude of material and child health problems ❑ Issues of maternal and child health: Age, gender, sexuality, psychosocio cultural factors ❑ Preventive obstetrics ❑ National health and family welfare programmes related to maternal and child health: health care delivery system—National Rural Health Mission, Role of NGO's ❑ Theories, models and approaches applied to midwifery practice ❑ Role and scope of midwifery practice: Independent nurse midwifery practitioner ❑ Legal and ethical issues: Code of ethics and standards of midwifery practice, standing orders ❑ Evidence based midwifery practice ❑ Research priorities in obstetric and gynecological nursing.
II	15	**Human reproduction** ❑ Review of anatomy and physiology of human reproductive system: male and female ❑ Hormonal cycles ❑ Embryology ❑ Genetics, teratology and counseling ❑ Clinical implications

I Year

III	25	**Pregnancy** ❑ Maternal adaptation: Physiological, psychosocial • Assessment—Maternal and fetal measures, maternal measures: History taking, examination—general, physical and obstetrical measure, identification of high risk, • Fetal measure-clinical parameters, biochemical-human estriol, maternal serum Alfa Feto-Protein, acetyl choline esterase (AchE), triple test aminocentesis, cordocentesis, chorionic villus sampling (CVS)), • Biophysical—(US imaging, fetal movement count, ultrasonography, cardiotocography, cardiotomography, nonstress test (NST), contraction stress test (CST), amnioscopy, fetoscopy, • Radiological examination, ❑ Interpretation of diagnostic tests and nursing implications ❑ Nursing management of the pregnant women, minor disorders of pregnancy and management, preparation for child birth and parenthood, importance of institutional delivery, choice of birth setting, importance and mobilizing of transportation, prenatal counseling, role of nurse and crisis intervention, identification of high risk pregnancy and refer ❑ Alternative/complementary therapies
IV	25	**Normal Labor and nursing management:** ❑ Essential factors of labor ❑ Stages and onset **First stage: Physiology of normal labor** • Use of partograph: Principles, use and critical analysis, evidence based studies • Analgesia and anesthesia in labor • Nursing management **Second stage** • Physiology, intrapartum monitoring • Nursing management. • Resuscitation, immediate newborn care and initiate breast feeding (Guidelines of National Neonatalogy Forum of India) **Third stage** • Physiology and nursing management **Fourth stage — Observation, critical analysis and nursing management.** • Various child birth practice: water birth, position change, etc. • Evidence based practice in relation to labor intervention **Role of nurse midwifery practitioner** • Alternative/complementary therapies
V	20	**Normal puerperium and nursing management** ❑ Physiology of puerperium ❑ Physiology of lactation, lactation management, exclusive breast feeding, baby friendly hospital initiative (BFHI) ❑ Assessment of postnatal women. ❑ Minor discomforts and complications of puerperium ❑ Management of mothers during puerperium: Postnatal exercises rooming in, bonding, warm chain ❑ Evidence based studies **Role of nurse midwifery practitioner** • Alternative/complementary therapies
VI	20	**Normal Newborn** ❑ Physiology and characteristics of normal newborn ❑ Physical and behavioral assessment of newborn ❑ Needs of newborn ❑ Essential newborn care: Exclusive breast feeding, immunization, hygiene measures, newborn nutrition ❑ Organization of neonatal care services (Levels), transport, neonatal intensive care unit, organization and management of nursing services in NICU ❑ Observation and care of newborn ❑ Parenting process

VII	10	**Pharmacodynamics in obstetrics** ❑ Drugs used in pregnancy, labor, postpartum and newborn ❑ Calculation of drug dose and administration ❑ Effects of drugs used ❑ Anesthesia and analgesia in obstetrics ❑ Role and responsibilities of midwifery nurse practitioner ❑ Standing orders and protocols and use of selected life saving drugs and interventions of obstetric emergencies approved by the MOHFW
VIII	10	**Family welfare services** ❑ Drugs used in pregnancy, labor, postpartum and newborn ❑ Calculation of drug dose and administration ❑ Effects of drugs used ❑ Anaesthesia and analygesia and obstetrics ❑ Roles and responsibilities of midwifery nurse practitioner ❑ Standing orders and protocols and use of selected life saving drugs and interventions of obstetric emergencies approved by the MOHFW
VIII	10	**Family welfare services** ❑ Population dynamics ❑ Demography trends: vital statistics, caloulation of indicators especially maternal and neonatal mortality rates and problems and other health problems ❑ Recent advancement in contraceptive technology ❑ Role of nurses in family welfare programes in all settings ❑ Role of independent nurse midwifery practitioner ❑ Family life education ❑ Evidence based studies ❑ Information, education and communication (IEC) ❑ Management information and evaluation system (MIES) ❑ Teaching and supervision of health team member
IX	5	**Infertility** ❑ Primary and secondary causes ❑ Diagnostic procedures ❑ Counseling: ethical and legal aspects of assisted reproductive technology (ART) ❑ Recent advancement in infertility management. ❑ Adoption procedures Role of nurses in infertility management
X	5	**Menopause** ❑ Physiological, psychological and social aspects ❑ Hormone replacement therapy ❑ Surgical menopause ❑ Counseling and guidance Role of midwifery nurse practitioner
XI	5	**Abortion** ❑ Types, causes ❑ Legislations, clinical rights and professional responsibility ❑ Abortion procedures ❑ Complications ❑ Nursing management Role of midwifery nurse practitioner

Practical

Total = 660 Hours
1 week = 30 Hours

S. No.	Department/Unit	No. of Week	Total Hours
1.	Antenatal wards and OPDs	4	120
2.	Labor room	5	150
3.	Postnatal ward	2	60
4.	Family planning clinics	2	60
5.	PHC/rural maternity settings	4	120
6.	Gynae	2	60
7.	Maternity OT	2	60
8.	NICU	1	30
	Total	**22 Weeks**	**660 Hours**

Procedures observed

- Diagnostic investigations: Amniocentesis, cordocentesis, chorionic villi sampling.
- Infertility management: Artificial reproduction: Artificial insemination, *in vitro* fertilization, and related procedures.

Procedures assisted

- Medical termination of pregnancy.

Procedures performed

- Antenatal assessment-20.
- Postnatal assessment-20.
- Assessment during labor: use of partograph - 20.
- Per vaginal examination-20.
- Conduct of normal delivery-20.
- Episiotomy and suturing-10.
- Setting up of delivery areas.
- Insertion of intrauterine devices (copper-T).

Others

- Identification of high risk women and referral.
- Health education: To women and their families.
- Motivation of couples for planned parenthood.

SPECIAL NOTES

CONTENTS FOR SPECIAL NOTES

Serial Number	Subject	Page Number
1.	Probable Signs of Pregnancy	711
2.	Presumptive Signs of Pregnancy	712
3.	Fundus Height at Various Weeks of Pregnancy	713
4.	Skin Changes in Pregnancy	714
5.	Physiological Changes of Pregnancy According to Trimester	715
6.	Discomforts of Pregnancy	716
7.	Leopold's Maneuvers	717
8.	Station or Degree of Engagement	718
9.	Fetal Position in Vertex Presentation	719
10.	Fetal Attitude	720
11.	Estimate the Degree of Effacement by Vaginal Examination	721
12.	Effacement and Dilatation of Cervix	722
13.	Position of Episiotomy Incision During Second Stage of Labor	723
14.	Mechanism of Normal Labor	724
15.	Time Intervals for Nursing Interventions During First Stage of Labor	725
16.	Time Intervals for Nursing Interventions During Second Stage of Labor	726
17.	Analgesics and Anesthetics used in Labor and Birth	727
18.	Postpartal Discharge Instructions	728
19.	Six Week Physical Assessment	729
20.	Danger Signs of Labor	731
21.	Types of Breech Presentation	732
22.	Transverse or Shoulder Presentation	733
23.	Vacuum Extraction Applied on Posterior Fontanel	734
24.	Breech Birth	735
25.	Forceps used for a Breech Birth	736
26.	Four Different Twin Presentations	737
27.	Assessing the Pregnant Woman with Complete Uterine Rupture	738
28.	Assessing the Effects of Trauma in the Pregnant Woman	739
29.	Assessing the Pregnant Adolescent for Risk Factors	740
30.	Assessing the Pregnant Woman over 40 Years for Complications	741
31.	Assessing the Pregnant Woman with Hypovolemic Shock	742
32.	Assessment of Pregnant Woman with Diabetes Mellitus	743
33.	Assessment of Pregnant Woman with Renal Disease	744
34.	Assessment of Pregnant Woman with Cardiac Disease	745
35.	Assessment of Pregnant Woman with Thromboembolic Disease	746
36.	Common Gynecologic Disorders	747
37.	Biochemical Test	749
38.	Amniocentesis	750
39.	Cordocentesis	751

Serial Number	Subject	Page Number
40.	Chorionic Villi Sampling	752
41.	Cryosurgery	753
42.	Kick Chart	754
43.	Standard Laboratory Values in Pregnancy	755
44.	Nursing Diagnosis in Obstetrics and Gynecology	757
45.	Theories in Midwifery Practice	759
46.	Nursing Research and Biostatistics	763

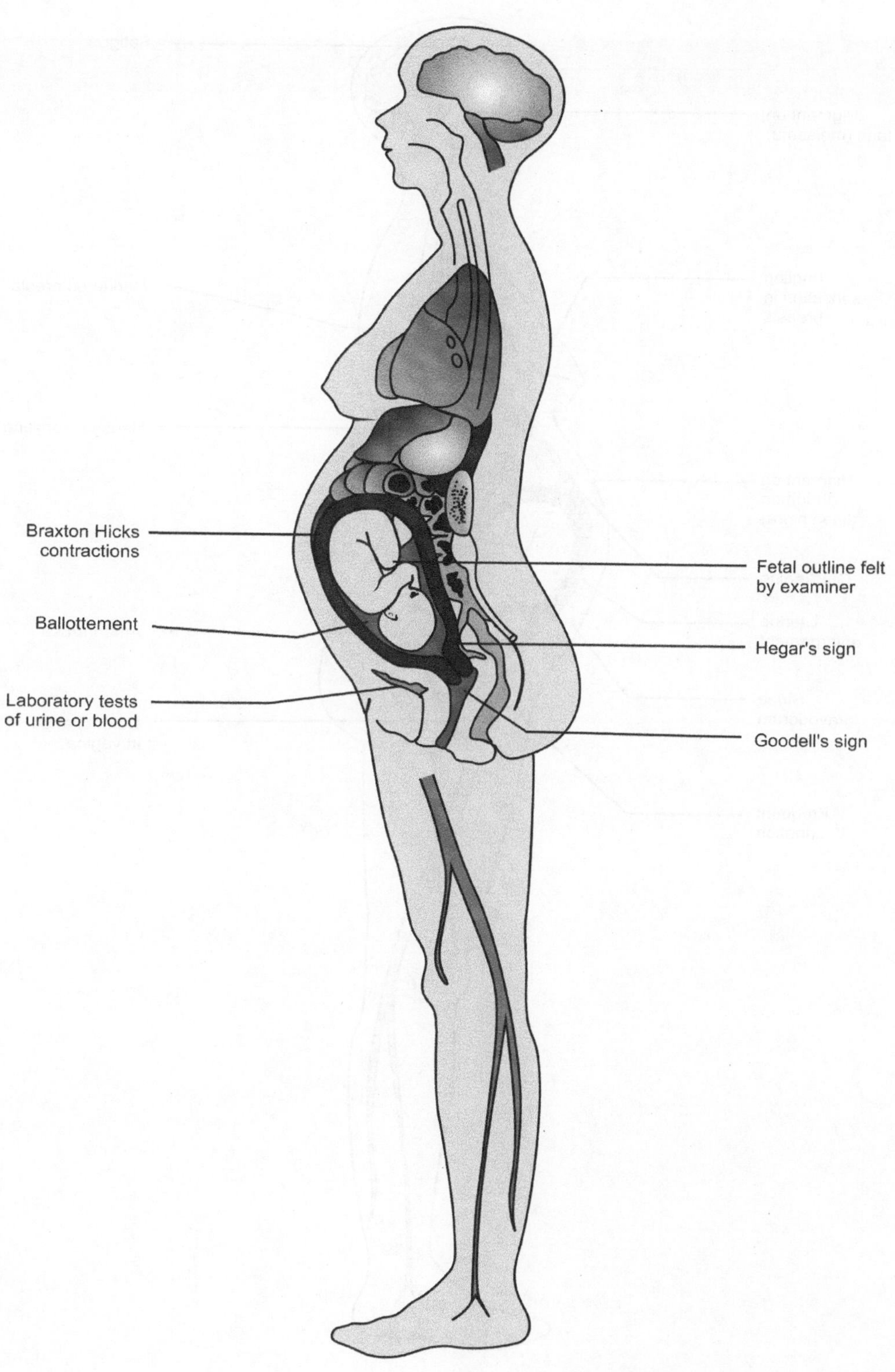
Braxton Hicks contractions
Ballottement
Laboratory tests of urine or blood
Fetal outline felt by examiner
Hegar's sign
Goodell's sign

PRESUMPTIVE SIGNS OF PREGNANCY

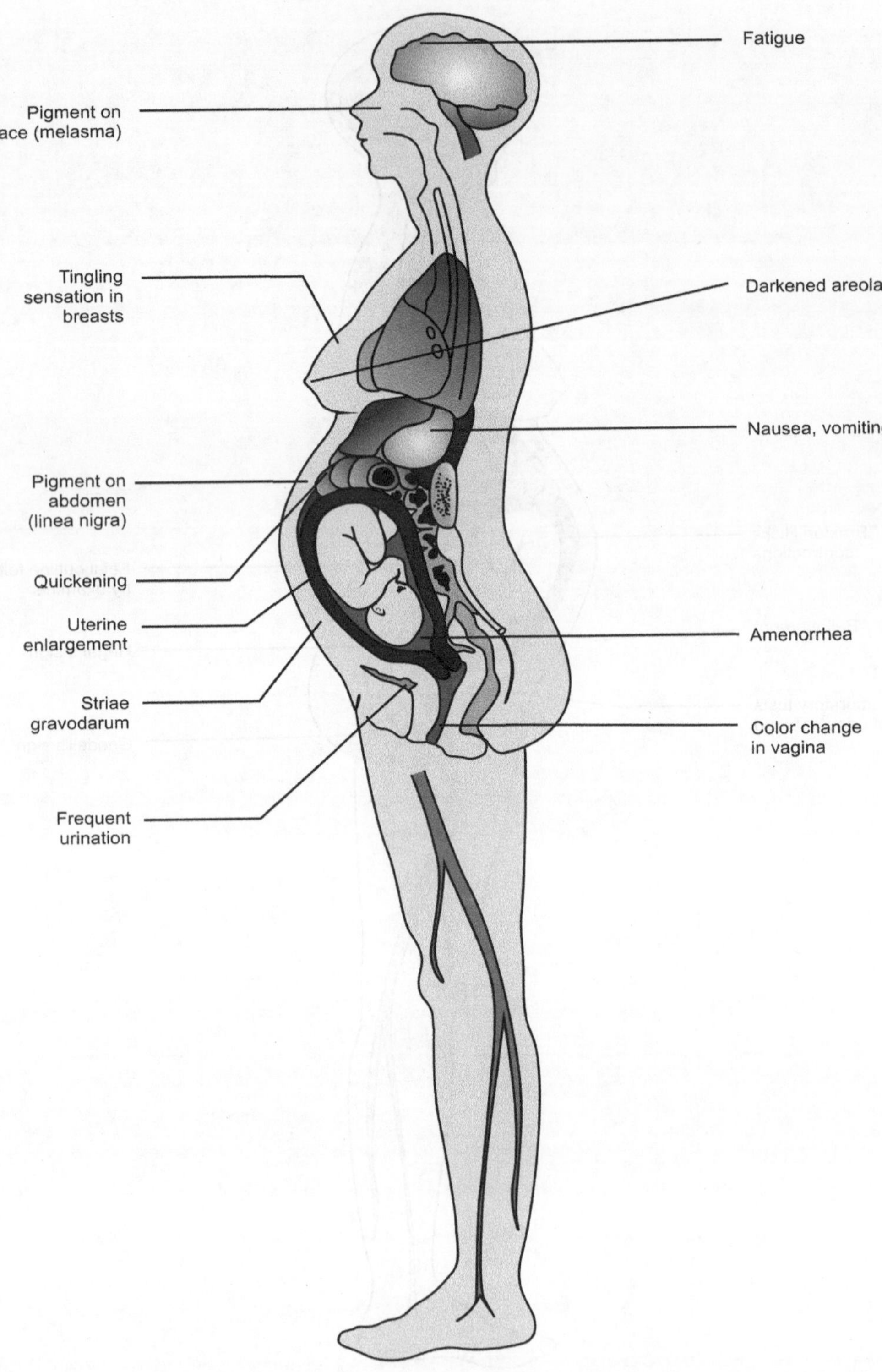

FUNDUS HEIGHT AT VARIOUS WEEKS OF PREGNANCY

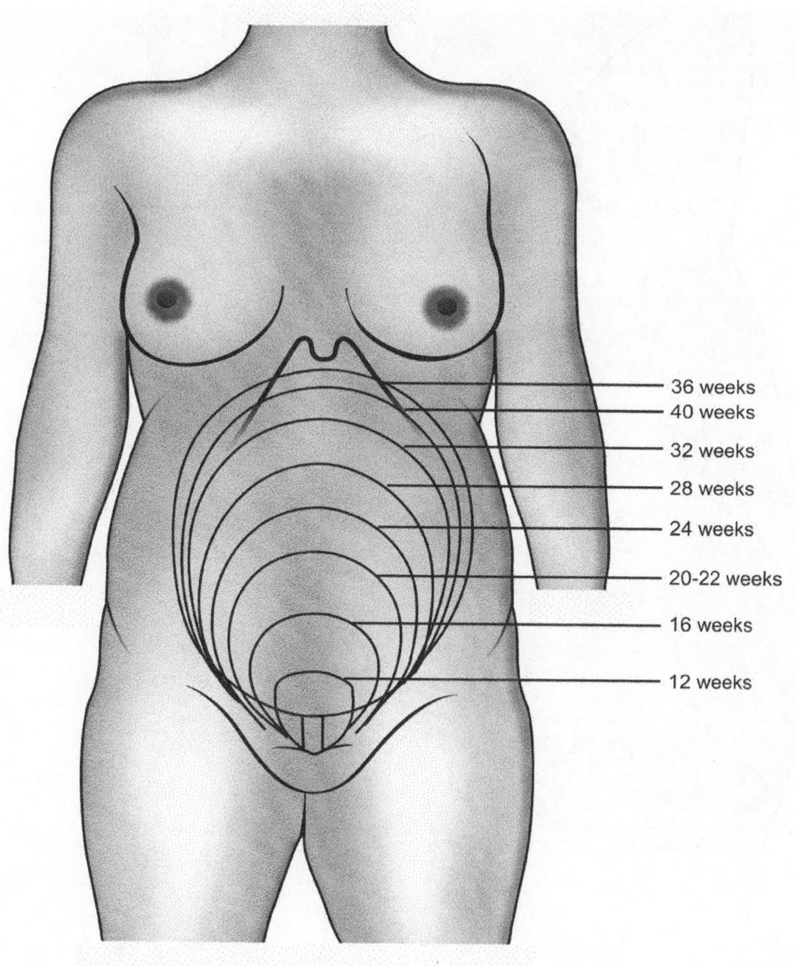

SKIN CHANGES IN PREGNANCY

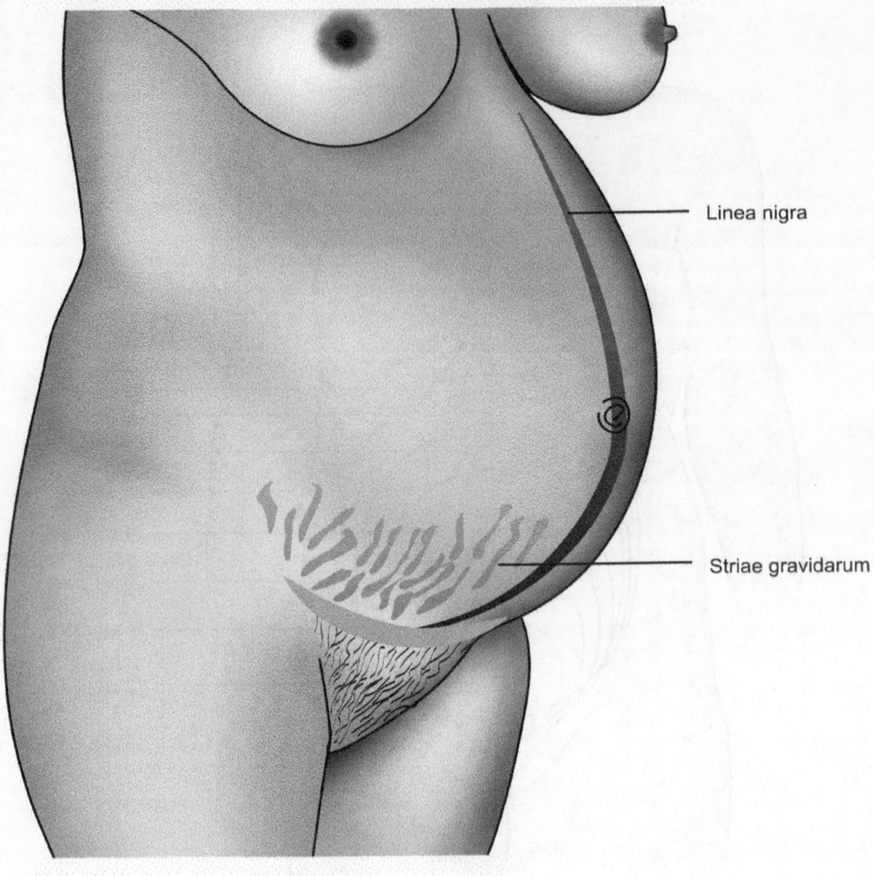

PHYSIOLOGICAL CHANGES OF PREGNANCY ACCORDING TO TRIMESTER

Location of Changes	Ist Trimester	IInd Trimester	IIIrd Trimester
Circulatory system	Blood volume increasing Pseudoanemia, clotting factors increasing	Blood pressure slightly decreased	Blood pressure return to prepregnancy level
Ovary	Corpus luteum active	Corpus luteum fading	
Uterus	Increased growth	Placenta forming estrogen and progesterone	
Cervix	Softening		Ripe increasing
Vagina	Progressive white discharge present		
Musculoskeletal system		Progressive cartilage softening Lordosis increasing	
Pigmentation		Progressively increasing	
Kidney	Maternal glomerular filteration rate increasing, Aldosterone increased, Retaining sodium and fluid	Glycosuria	
Gastrointestinal system			Slowed peristalsis
Thyroid	Increased metabolic rate		

DISCOMFORTS OF PREGNANCY

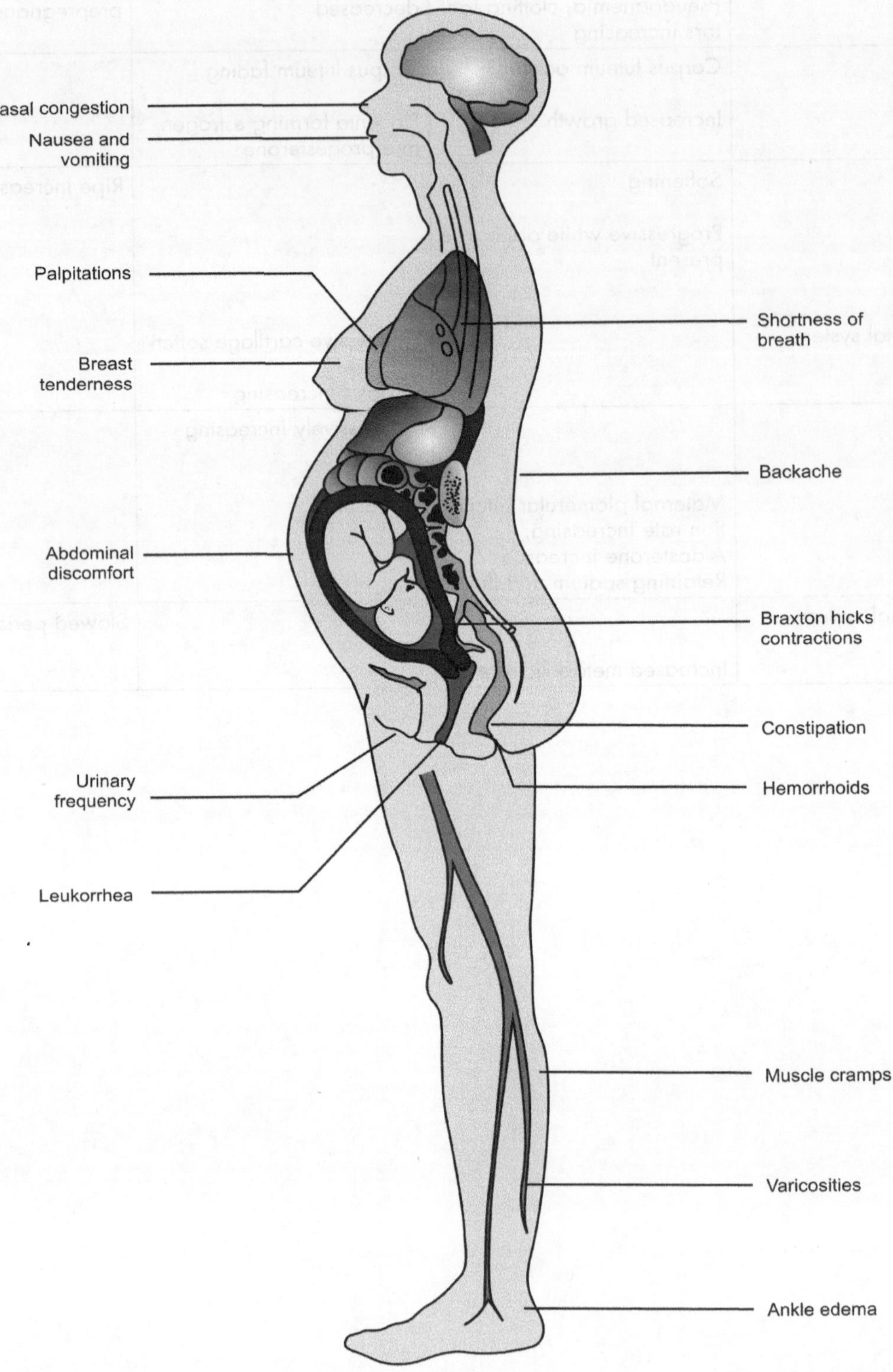

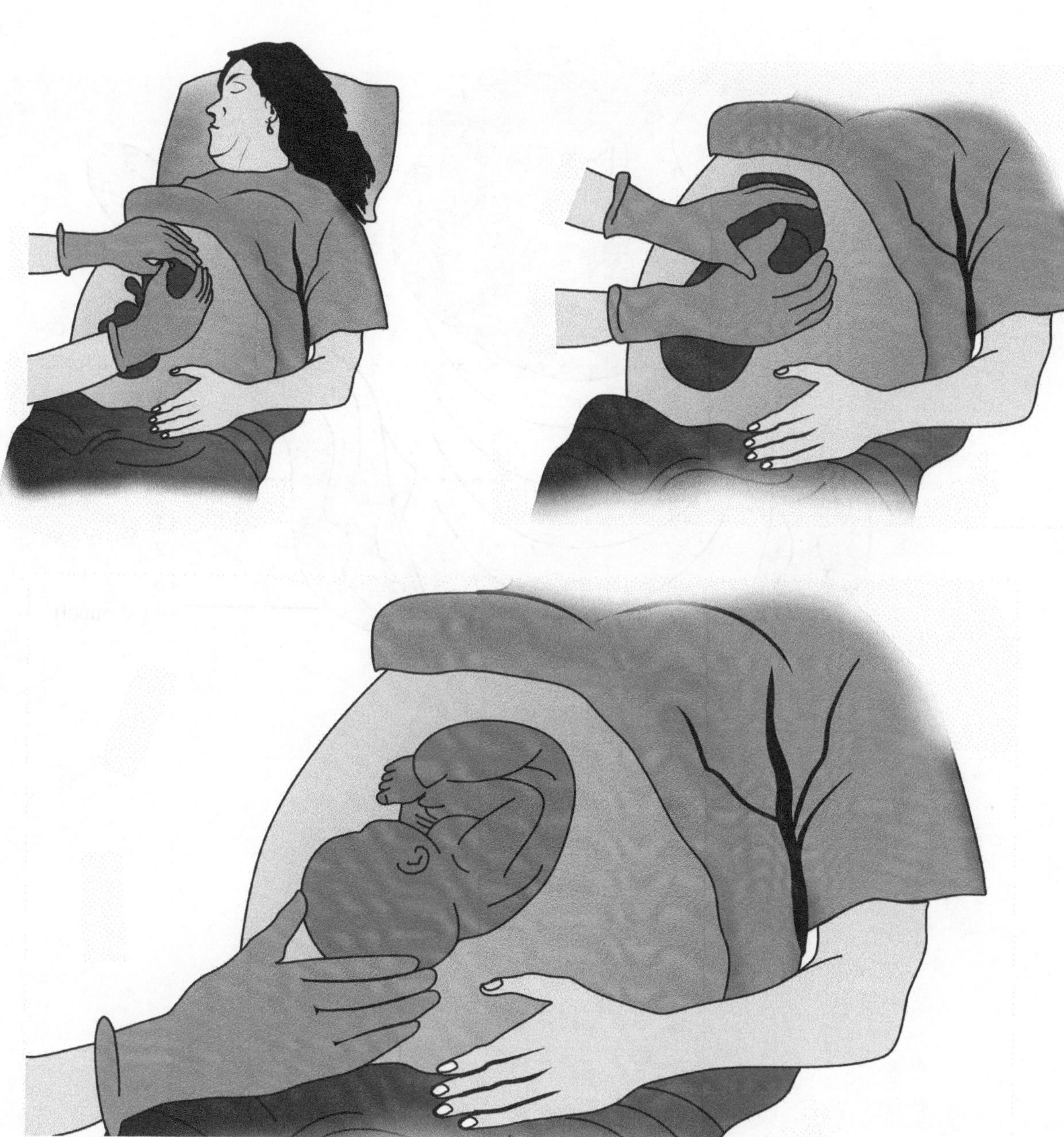

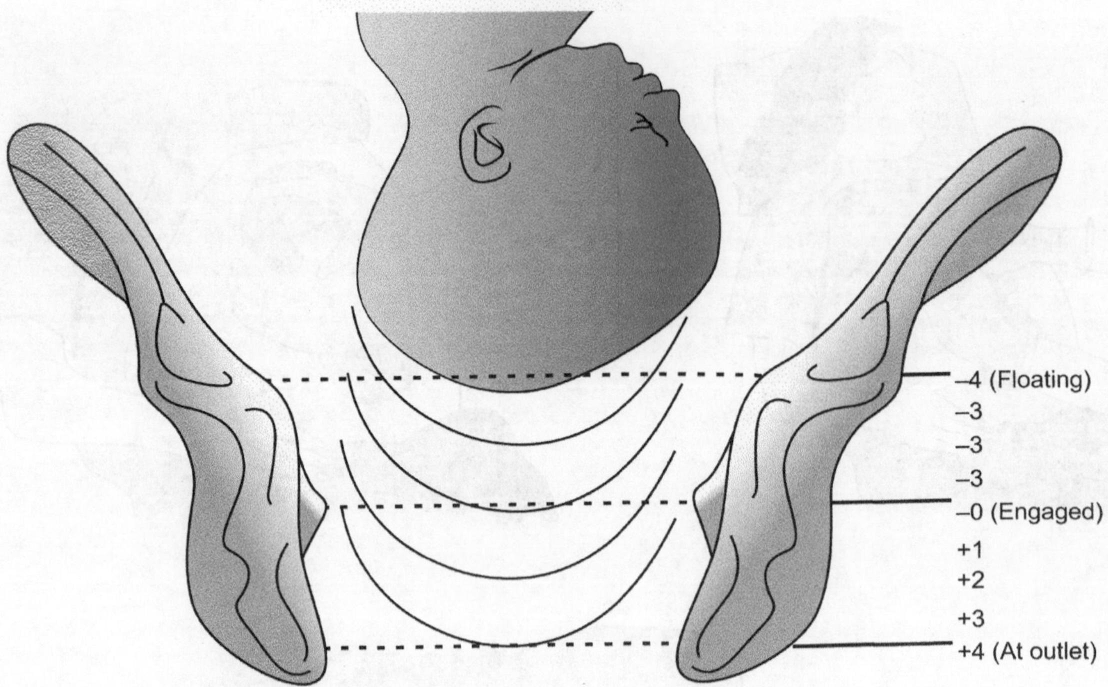
–4 (Floating)
–3
–3
–3
–0 (Engaged)
+1
+2
+3
+4 (At outlet)

FETAL POSITION IN VERTEX PRESENTATION

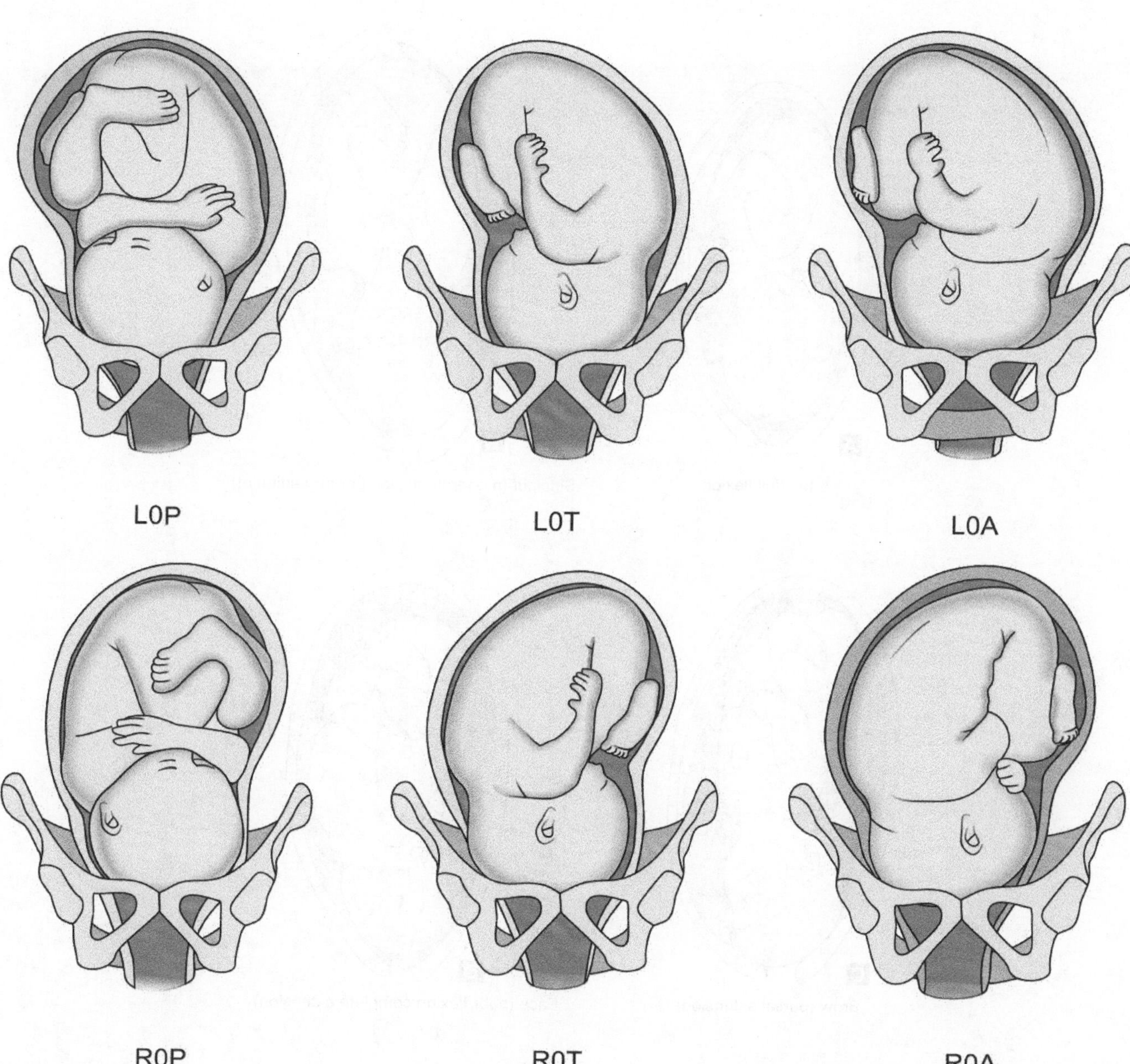

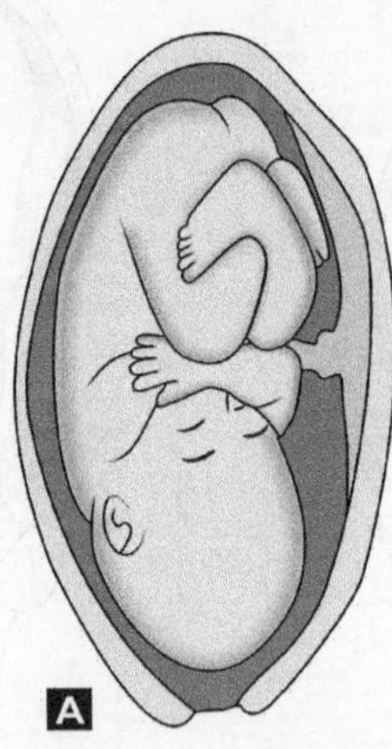

Vertex (full flexion)

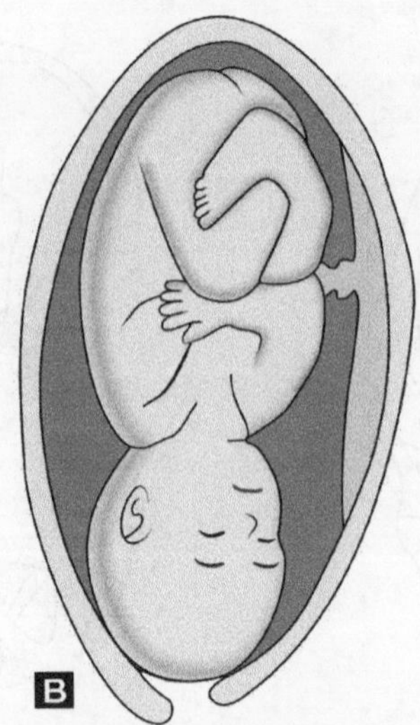

Sinciput (moderate flexion [military attitude])

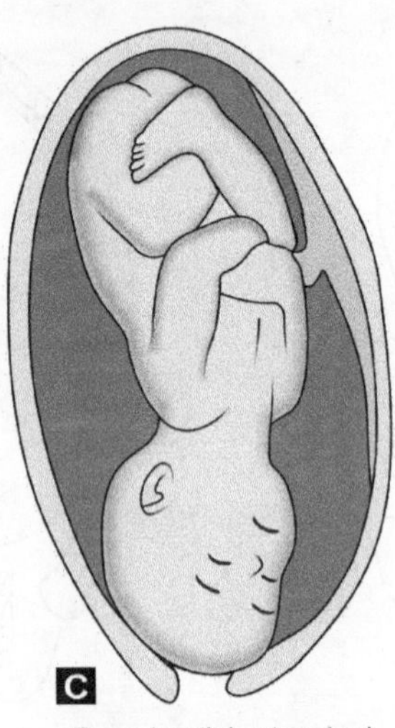

Brow (partial extension)

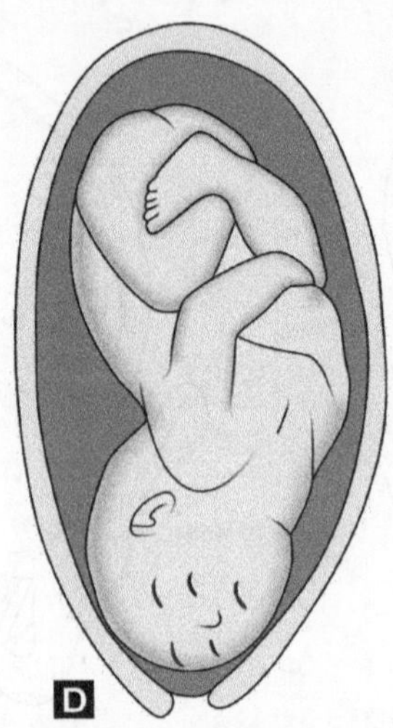

Face (poor flexion,complete extension)

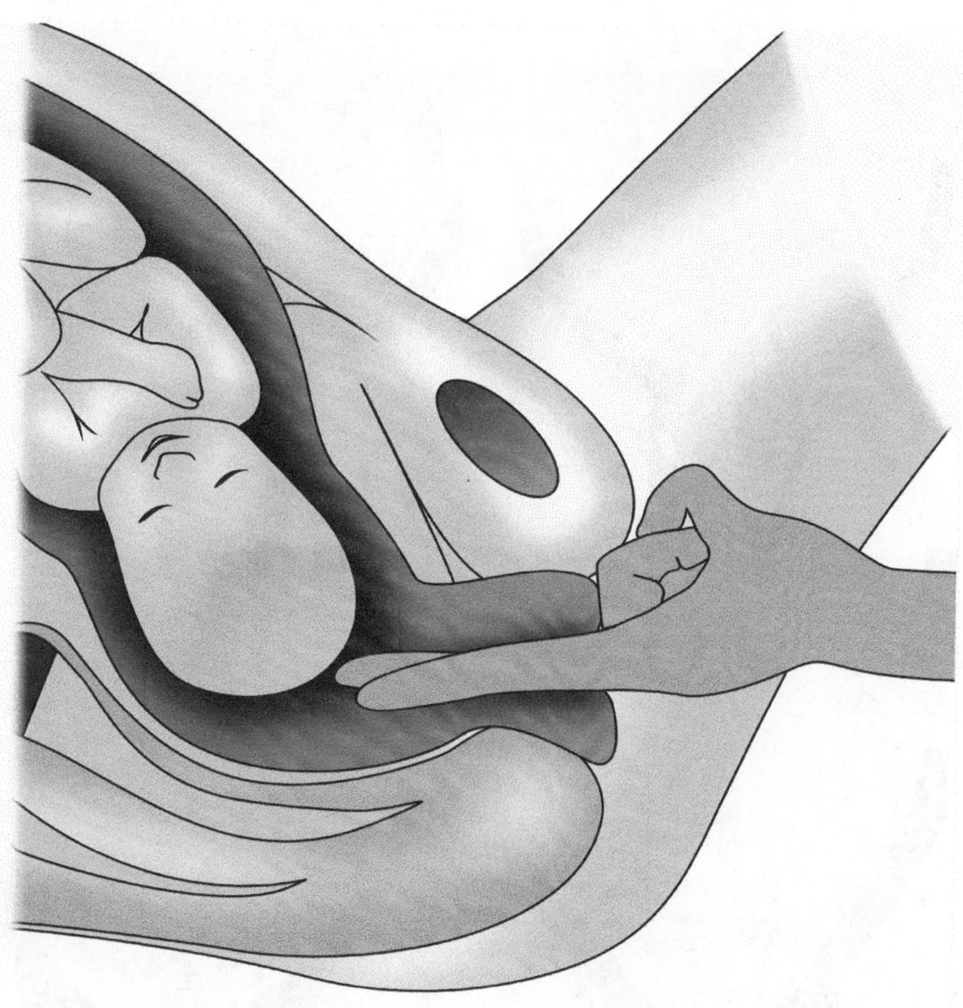

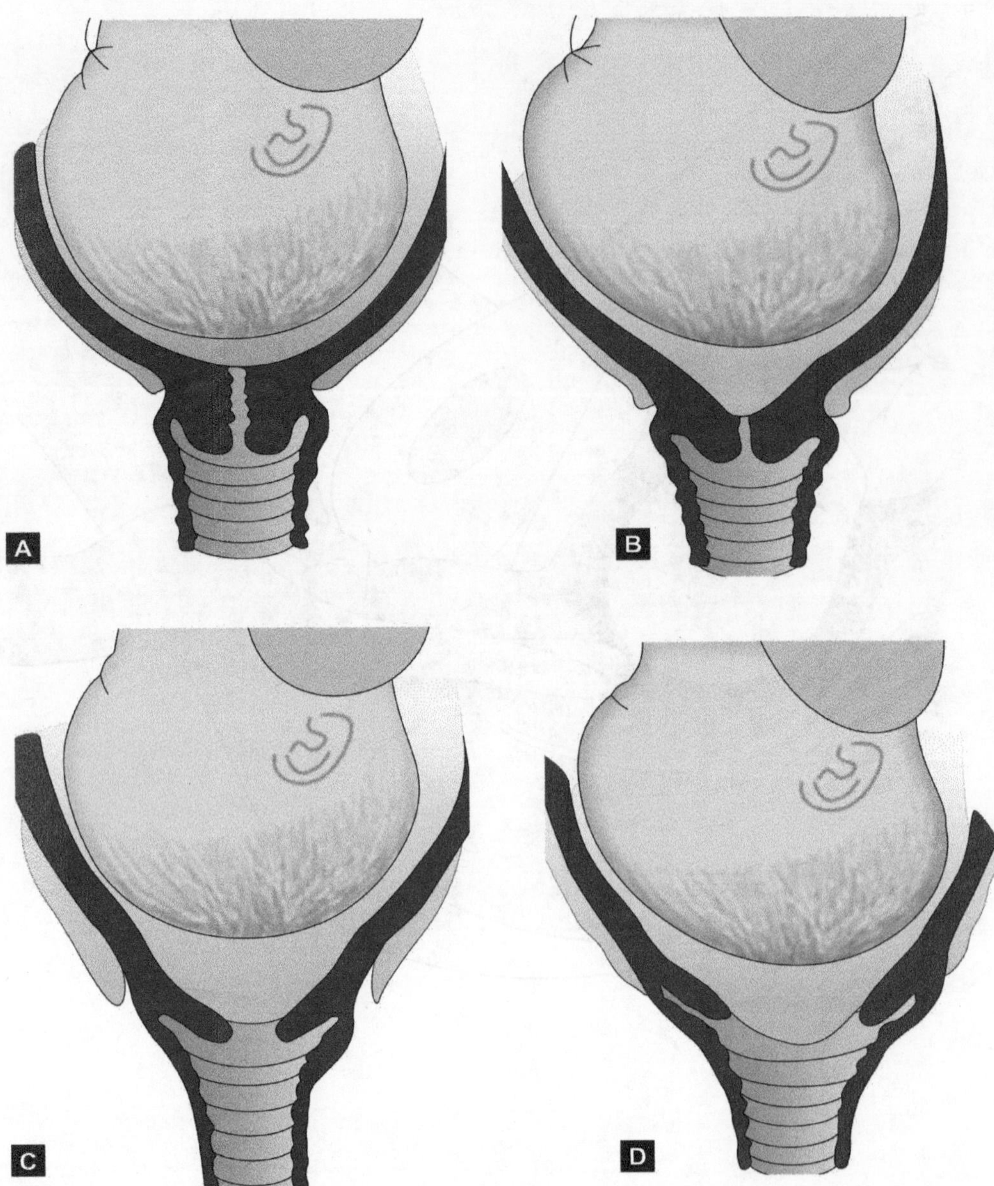
A
B
C
D

POSITION OF EPISIOTOMY INCISION DURING SECOND STAGE OF LABOR

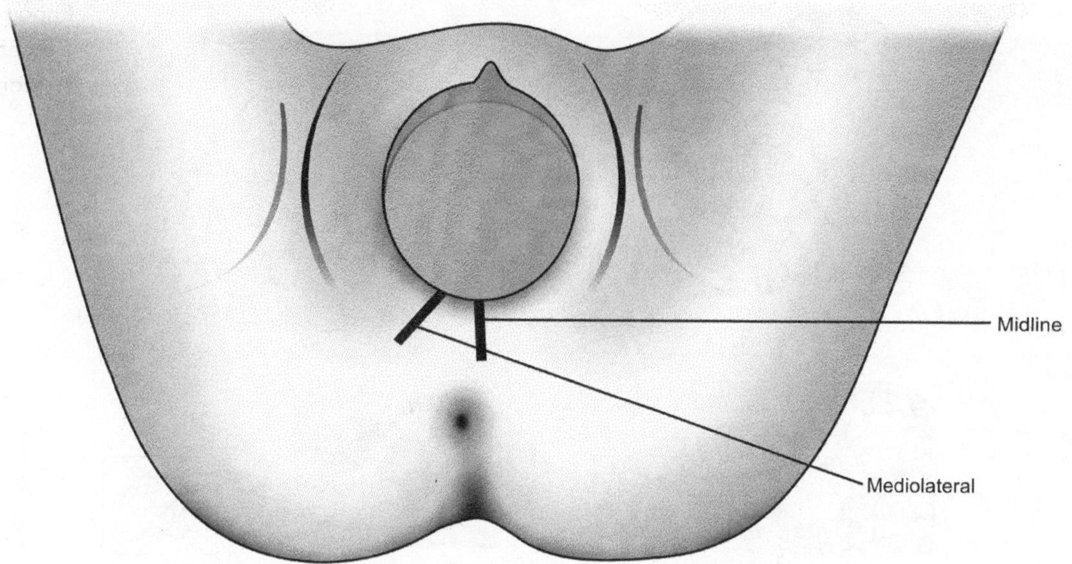

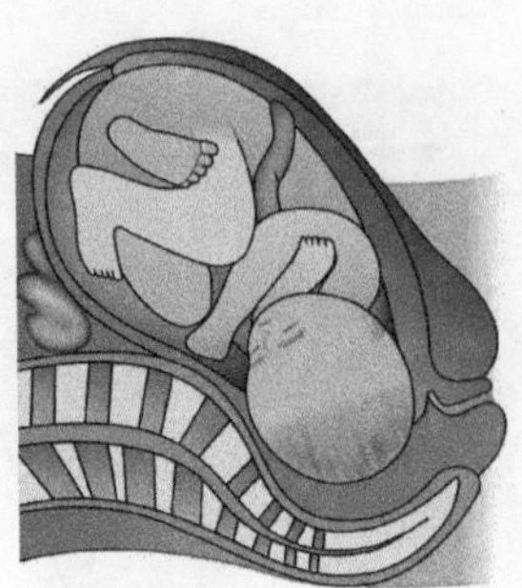

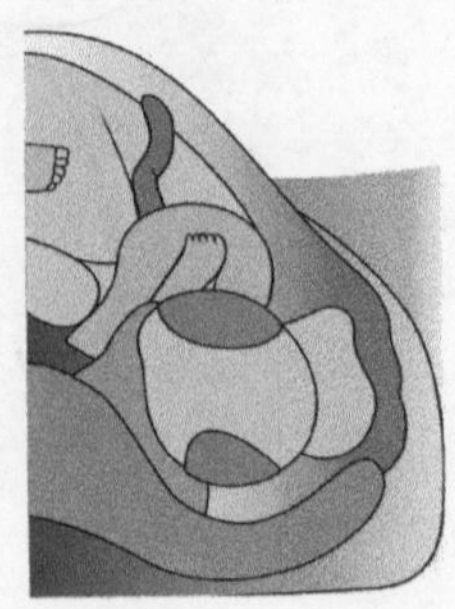

Engagement, Descent, Flexion

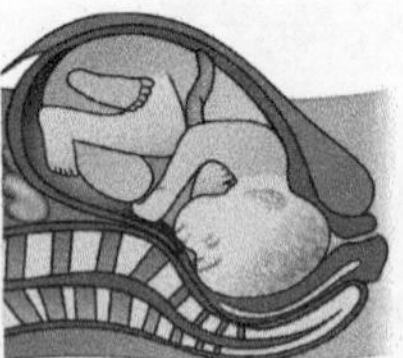

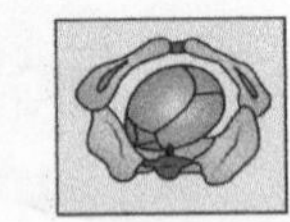

Internal rotation

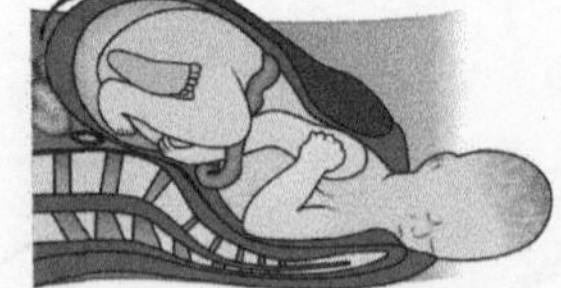

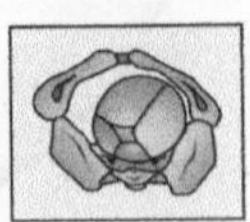

External rotation (restitution)

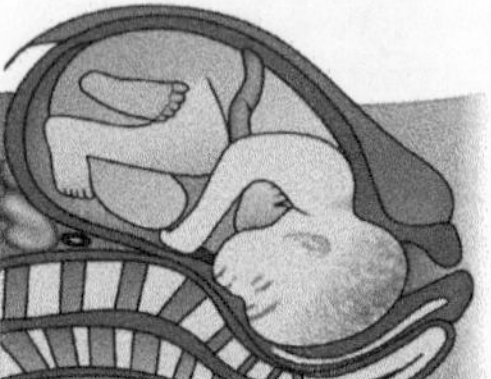

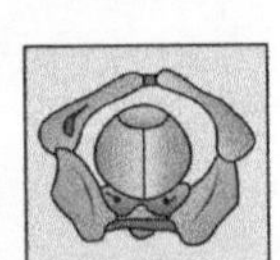

Extension beginning (rotation complete)

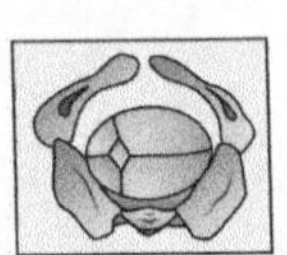

External rotation (shoulder rotation)

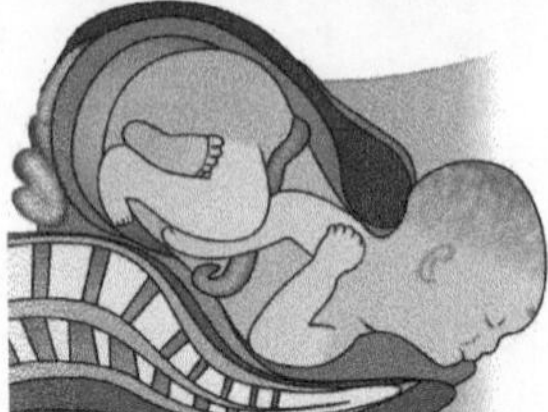

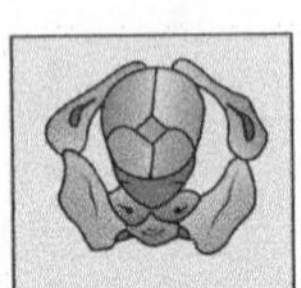

Extension complete

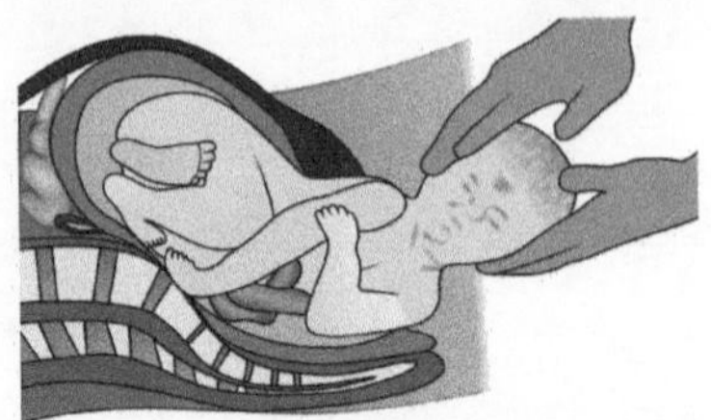

Expulsion

TIME INTERVALS FOR NURSING INTERVENTIONS DURING FIRST STAGE OF LABOR

Intervention	Assessment on Admission	Latent Phase [0-3 cm]	Active Phase [4-7 cm]	Transition Phase [8-10 cm]
Assess and record temperature	X	Q4hr[unless membranes are ruptured, then q2hr]	Q4hr[unless membranes are ruptured, then q2hr]	Q4hr[unless membranes are ruptured, then q2hr]
Pulse	X	q30-60 min	q30-60 min	q15-30 min
Respiration	X	q30-60 min	q30-60 min	q15-30 min
Blood pressure	X	q30-60 min	q30-60 min	q15-30 min
Voiding	X	q2 hr	q2 hr	q2 hr
FHR	X	Continuous monitor or q30-60 min	Continuous monitor or Q15-30 min	Continuous monitor or Q15-30 min
Contractions	X	Continuous monitor or q30-60 min	Continuous monitor or Q15-30 min	Continuous monitor or Q15-30 min
Perineum	X	q30-60 min	q30 min	Q15 min
Provide ambulation	X	Until membrane rupture	Until membrane rupture	
Support	X	continuously	continuously	continuously

TIME INTERVALS FOR NURSING INTERVENTIONS DURING SECOND STAGE OF LABOR

Intervention	Beginning of 2nd Stage	Continued Frequency	After Birth of Infant	After Delivery of Placenta
Assess and record temperature	X	q2 hr		q1 hr
Pulse	X	q1 hr	X	q15 min
Respiration	X	q5-30 min	X	q15 min
Blood pressure	X	q5-30 min	x	x
FHR	X	continuous monitor or q5 min		
Contractions	X	continuous monitor or q5 min		
Perineum	X	q15 min		q15 min
Provide Support	x	continuously	continuously	continuously

ANALGESICS AND ANESTHETICS USED IN LABOR AND BIRTH

Type	Drug	Dose/Route	Effect on Mother	Effect on Labor Progress	Effect on Betus or Bew Born
Narcotic analgesics	Meperidine [Demerol]	25 mg IV 50-100 mg IM q3-4hr, also epidurally	Effective analgesic: Feeling of well being	Relaxation, possibly aiding progress during cervical relaxation. Slows labor contractions if given early.	Should be given 3 hr before birth to avoid respiratory depression in new born. Decreases beat to beat variability in FHR.
	Nalbuphine [Nubain]	10-20mg IM q3-6 hr, 0.3-3 mg/kg over 10-15 minIV	Slowing of respiratory rate; effective analgesic	Mild maternal sedation	Results in some respiratory depression
	Butorphanol [Stadol]	1-2 mg IM or IV q3-4 hr	Withdrawal symptoms if woman is opiate dependent	Possible slowing of labor if given early	Results in some respiratory depression
	Morphine sulfate	Intrathecally 0.2-1mg 5mg epidurally	Pruritus; effective analgesia	Possible slowing of labor contractions	some respiratory depression
	Fentanyl [Sublimaze]	50-100 μg IM or 25-50 μgIV; also epidurally	Hypotension; Respiratory depression	Slowing of labor if given early	May result in respiratory depression
Lumbar epidural block	Local anesthetic Bupivacaine [Marcaine] Ropivacaine [Naropin]	Administered for first stage of labor; with continuous block, anesthesia will last through birth;injected at L3-4; fentanyl or morphine possibly added	Rapid onset,inminutes;lasting 60-90 min;loss of pain perception for labor contractions and birth; possible maternal hypo tension	Slowing of labor if given early; pushing feeding obliterated,resulting in possible prolonged second stage .	May be some differences in response in first few days of life .
Pudendal block	Local anesthetic lidocaine [Xylocaine]	Administered just before birth for perineal anesthesia; injected through vagina	Rapid anesthesia of perineum	None apparent	None apparent
Local infilteration of perineum	Local anesthetic lidocaine [Xylocaine]	Injected just before episiotomy incision	Anesthesia of perineum almost immediately	None apparent	None apparent
General intravenous anesthetics	Thiopental	Administered by anesthesiologist or nurse anesthetist	Rapid anesthesia;also rapid recovery	Forceps required because abdominal pushing is no longer.	Results in infant being born with CNS depression

POSTPARTAL DISCHARGE INSTRUCTIONS

Topic	Instructions
Work	All women should avoid heavy work for at least the first 3 weeks after birth. Women differ in their concept of heavy work, so it is a good idea to explore what a woman considers heavy work. It is usually advised that a woman not return to an outside job for at least 3 weeks not only for her own health but also for enjoyment of the early weeks with her new born.
Rest	A woman should plan at least one rest period each day and try to get a good night's sleep. She can rest during the day when her newborn is sleeping, unless she has other children or an aged parent to care for. If she has others dependent on her explore the possibility of having a neighbor, another family member or a person from a community health agency relieve her.
Exercise	A woman should limit the number of stairs she climbs to one flight/day for the first week at home. Beginning the second week, it her lochial discharge is normal, she may start to increase this activity. This limitation will involve some planning on her part. She should continue with muscle strengthening exercise such as abdominal crunches.
Hygiene	A woman may take tub bath or showers. She should continue to apply any cream or ointment as ordered for the perineal area and cleanse her perineum from front to back. Any perineal stitches will be absorbed within 10 days. She should not use vaginal douches until she returns for her postpartal check up.
Coitus	It is safe as soon as a woman's lochia has turned to alba and, if present, episiotomy is healed. Use of lubricating jelly will aid comfort because vaginal cells may not be as thick as formerly because pregnancy hormone balance has not yet completely returned.
Contraception	If desired, a woman should begin a contraception measure with the initiation of coitus. If she wishes an IUD, this may be fitted immediately after birth or at her first postpartal checkup. Oral contraceptives are begun about 2-3 weeks after birth. A diaphragm must be refitted at a 6 week checkup. Until she returns for this checkup, an over the counter spermicidal jelly and condoms can provide protection.
Follow-up	A woman should notify her physician or nurse-midwife if she notices an increase, not a decrease, in lochial discharge, or if lochia serosa or lochia alba becomes lochia rubra. Delayed postpartal hemorrhage can occur in women who become extremely fatigued. Getting adequate rest during her first weeks at home will do much to prevent the possibility of this complication. 4 to 6 weeks after birth, a woman should return to her physician or nurse midwife for an examination. This visit is important to ensure that involution is complete, immunization against the virus associated with cervical cancer (HPV), and reproductive life planning.

SIX WEEK PHYSICAL ASSESSMENT

HISTORY

Assess the chief concern, family profile (support, system, bonding, self esteem, and family integrity), interval history, and review of systems (urinary system for pain, frequency, or stress incontinence along with gastrointestinal tract and reproductive tract in particular).

Assess maternal intake. Some new mothers are too to eat well, so they eat mainly carbohydrate snack foods, or, atleast, not a balanced diet.

PHYSICAL EXAMINATION

General Appearance

Alert; positive mood. If not, woman is probably still extremely fatigued.

Weight

Achievement of pre-pregnant weight; if not, this will be her baseline post-pregnant weight.

Hair

Healthy, firm hair; excess loss of hair from early postpartum period has halted

Eyes

Pink and moist conjunctiva; if pallor persists, diet may be inadequate because of fatigue.

Breasts

Nursing Woman: Full and firm to palpation; blue veins prominent under skin; only slightly tender. No palpable nodules or lumps. If erythematous or tender, mastitis may be present. If fessures on nipples are present, the woman may need to expose her nipples to air or to apply additional cream. An occasional filled milk gland may present as lump; re-examine after breast feeding.

Non-nursing Woman: Return to pre-pregnant size; no palpable nodules or lumps.

Abdomen

Striae less prominent; linea nigra fading, muscle tone improving. No distended bowel from constipation. No distended bladder from retention. No history of pain, frequency, or blood on urination. If lax abdominal muscle tone is present, women need to increase fluid and fiber. Urinary symptoms probably reflect urinary infection (that needs specific treatment).

Parineum and Uterus

No lochia; cervix closed; uterus has returned to pre-pregnant size—pap test is normal. Ask woman to bear down during pelvic examination to observe for uterine prolapsed, rectocele, or cystocele. If involution is not complete; reason for sub involution must be investigated.

Lower Extremities

Varicosities barely noticeable.

Rectum

Hemorrhoids receded to pre-pregnant size or are no longer observable.

LABORATORY REPORT

Hematocrit = 37% Hemoglobin = 11-12g/100 ml

If these are low, reassess diet; possibly iron supplement may be needed.

Rubella antibody titer = 1:8

If low, additional immunization is recommended before a second pregnancy.

IMMUNIZATION STATUS

Assess need for human papillomavirus (HPV) or rubella vaccine.

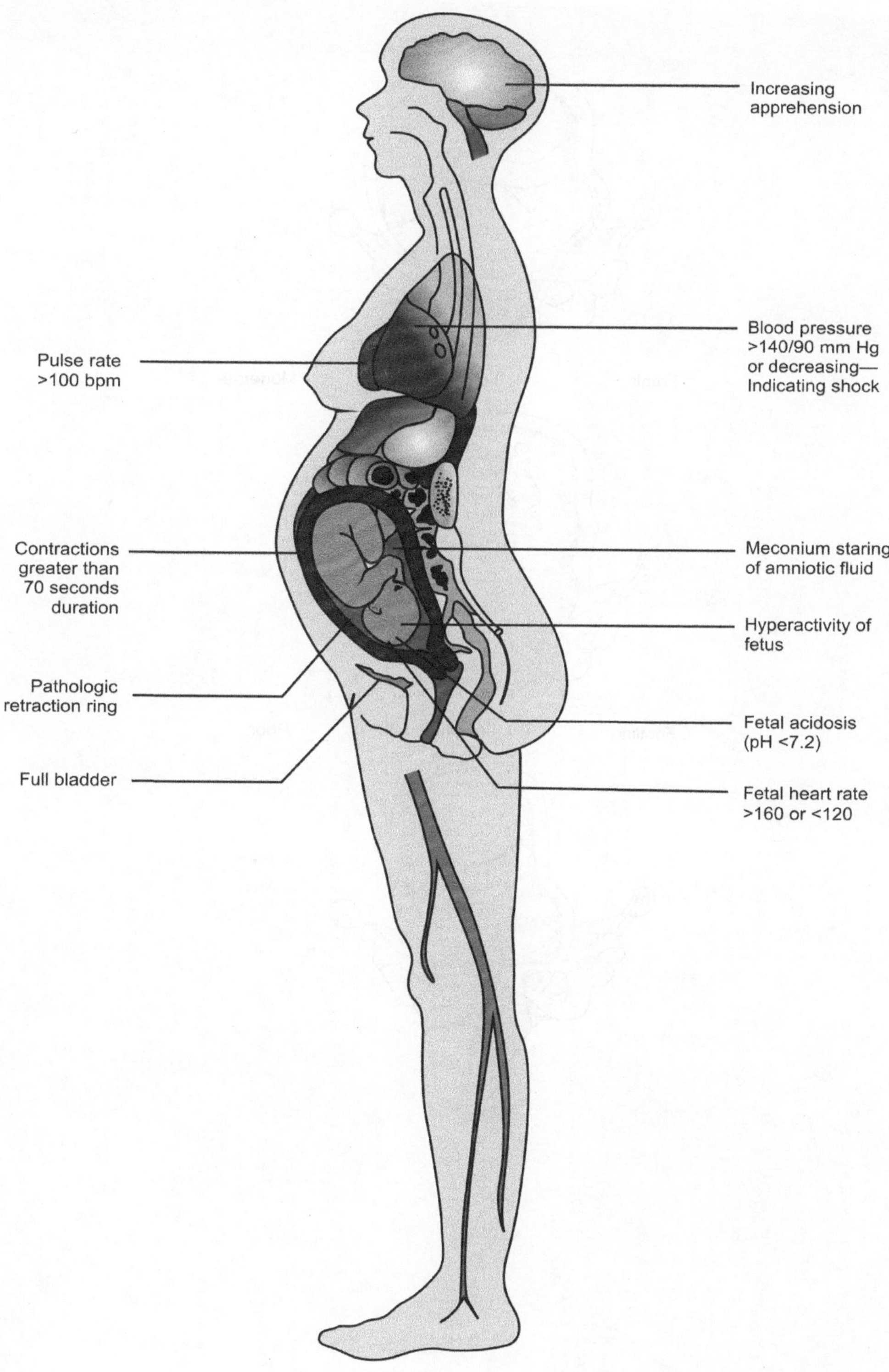
Increasing
apprehension
Blood pressure
>140/90 mm Hg
or decreasing—
Indicating shock
Pulse rate
>100 bpm
Contractions
greater than
70 seconds
duration
Meconium staring
of amniotic fluid
Hyperactivity of
fetus
Pathologic
retraction ring
Fetal acidosis
(pH <7.2)
Full bladder
Fetal heart rate
>160 or <120

Complete type longitudinal lie good attitude

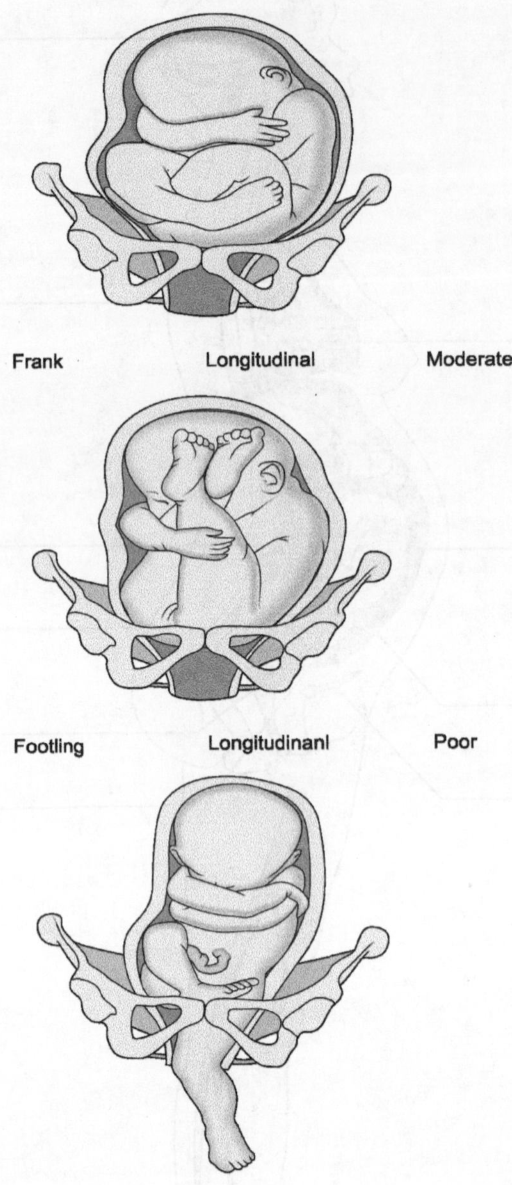

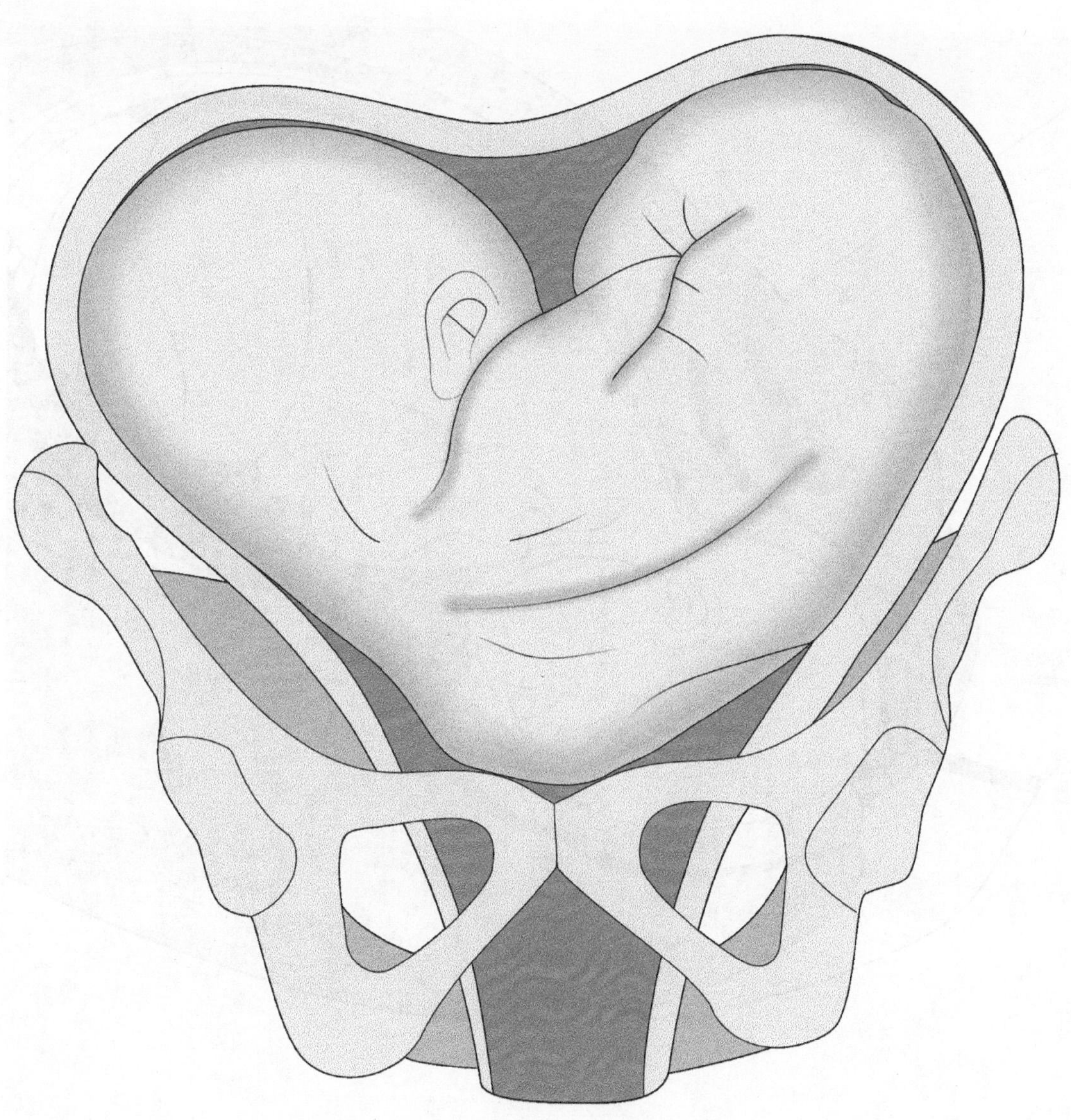

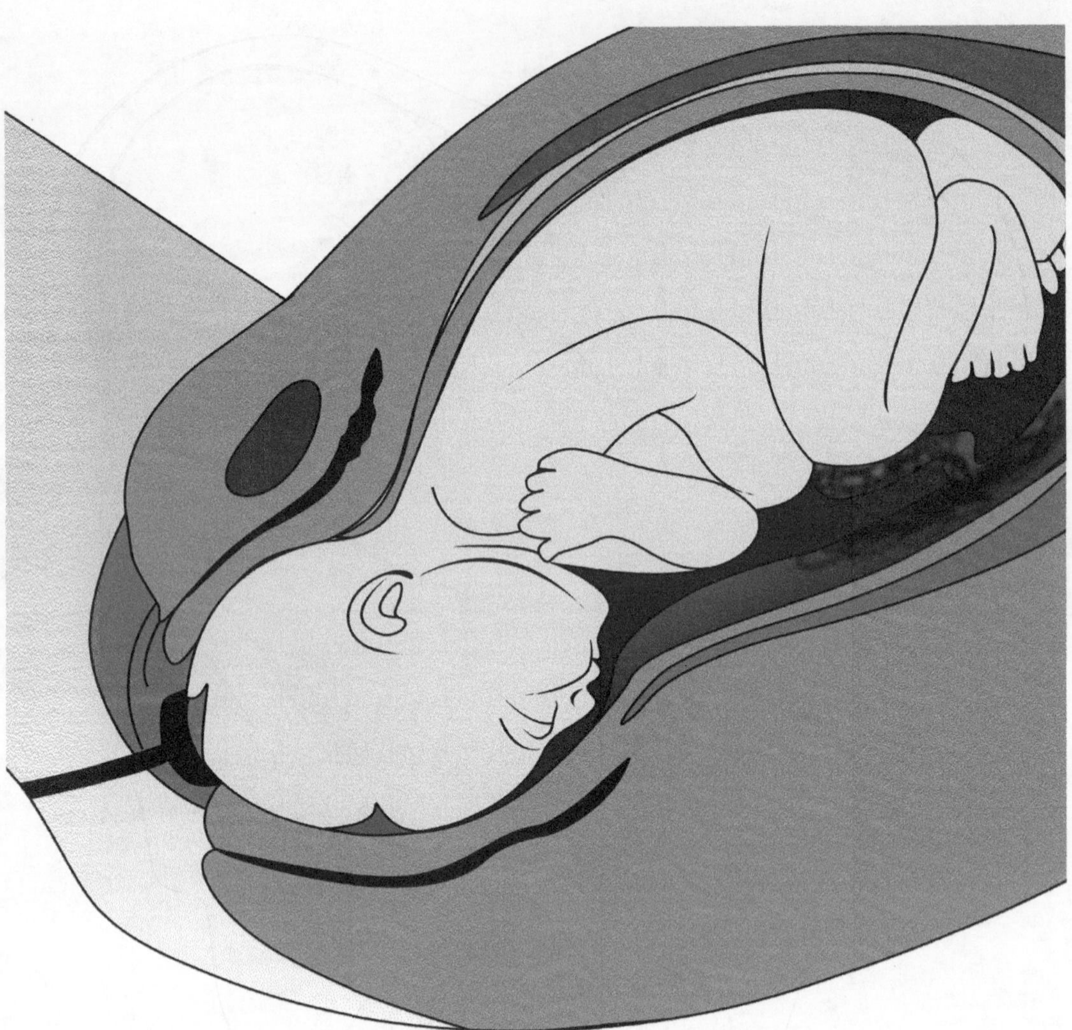

BREECH BIRTH

A. Position before labor; left sacroposterior

B. Descent and internal rotation

C. Legs being born; the shoulders turn to present to the anteroposterior diameter

D. The head is born.

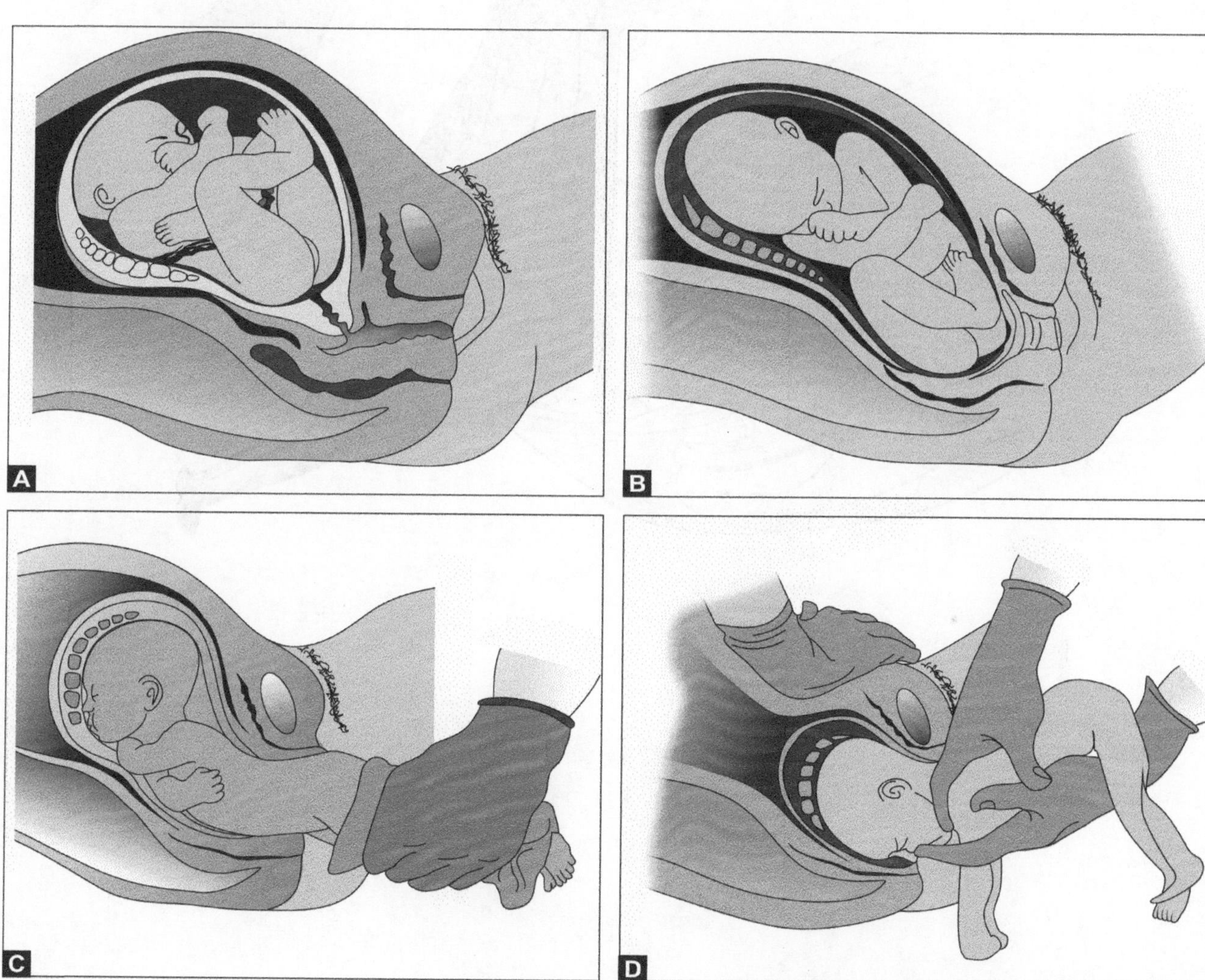

FORCEPS USED FOR A BREECH BIRTH

Traction is applied directly to the head, so damage to the infant's neck is avoided.

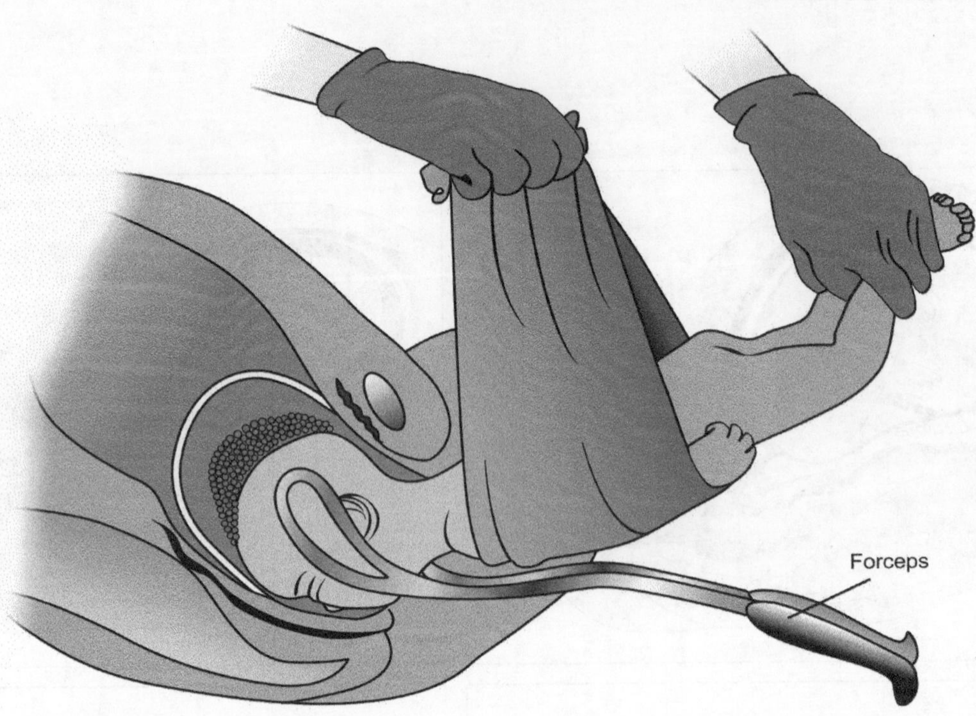

FOUR DIFFERENT TWIN PRESENTATIONS

A. Both infant vertex

B. One infant vertex and one breech

C. Both infants breech

D. One infant vertex and one in transverse.

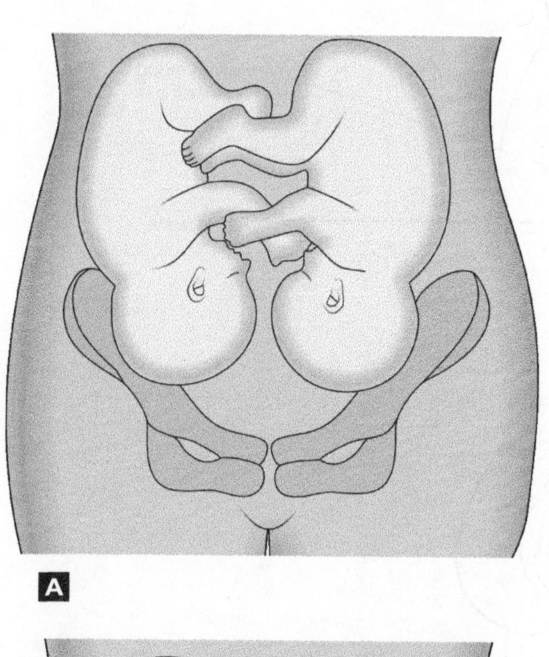

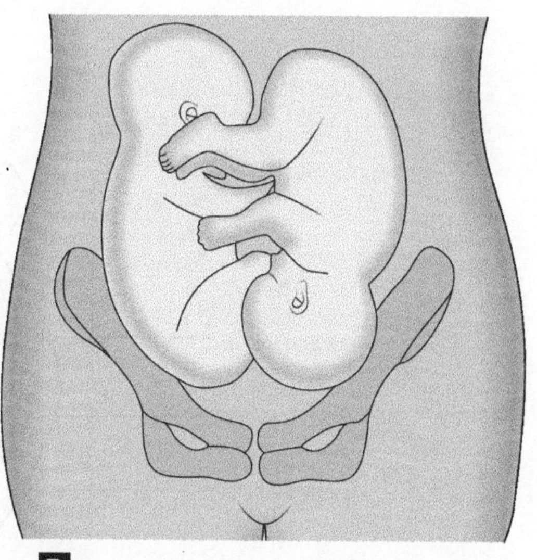

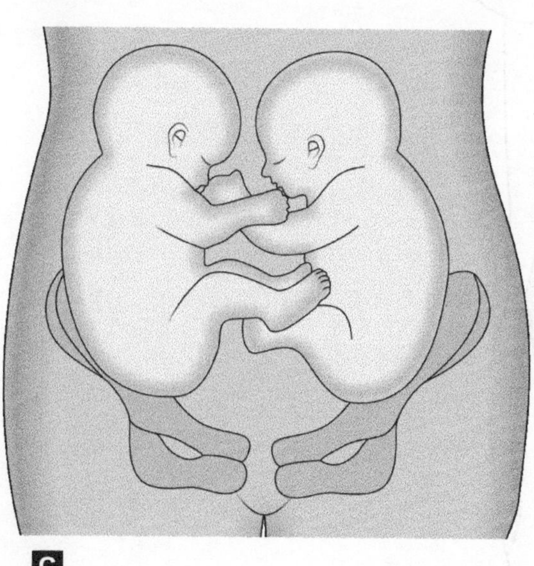

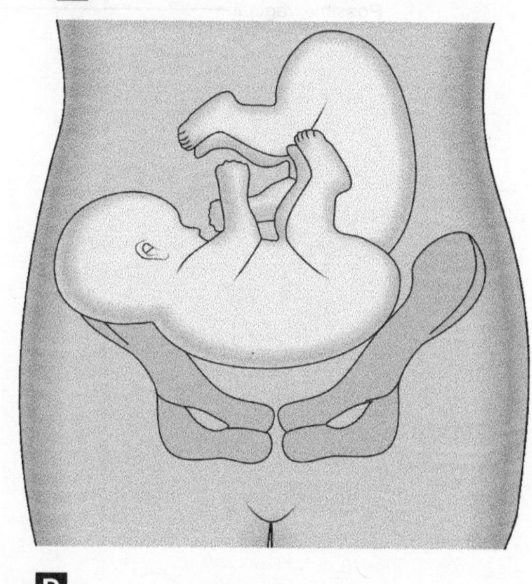

ASSESSING THE PREGNANT WOMAN WITH COMPLETE UTERINE RUPTURE

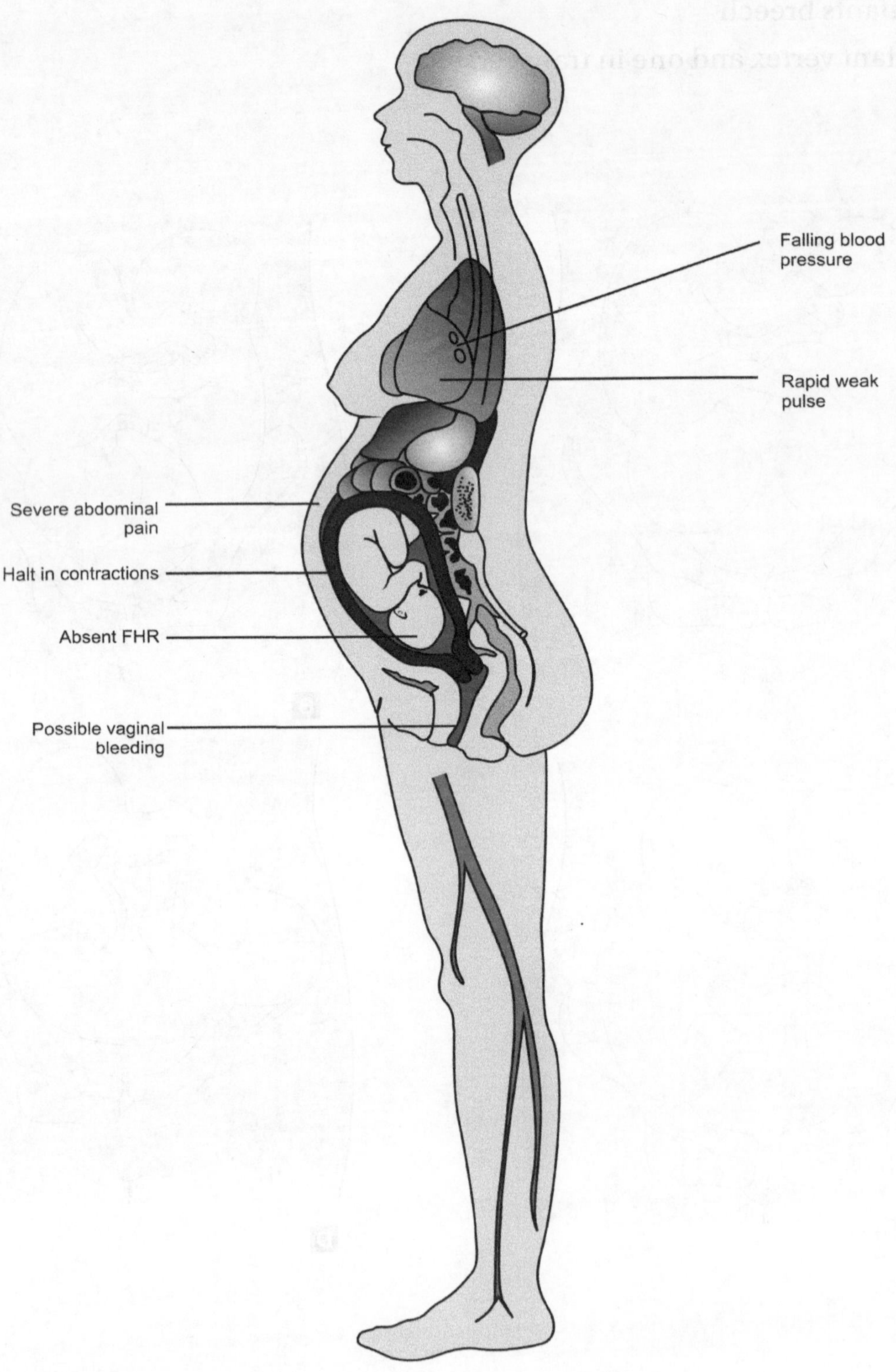

ASSESSING THE EFFECTS OF TRAUMA IN THE PREGNANT WOMAN

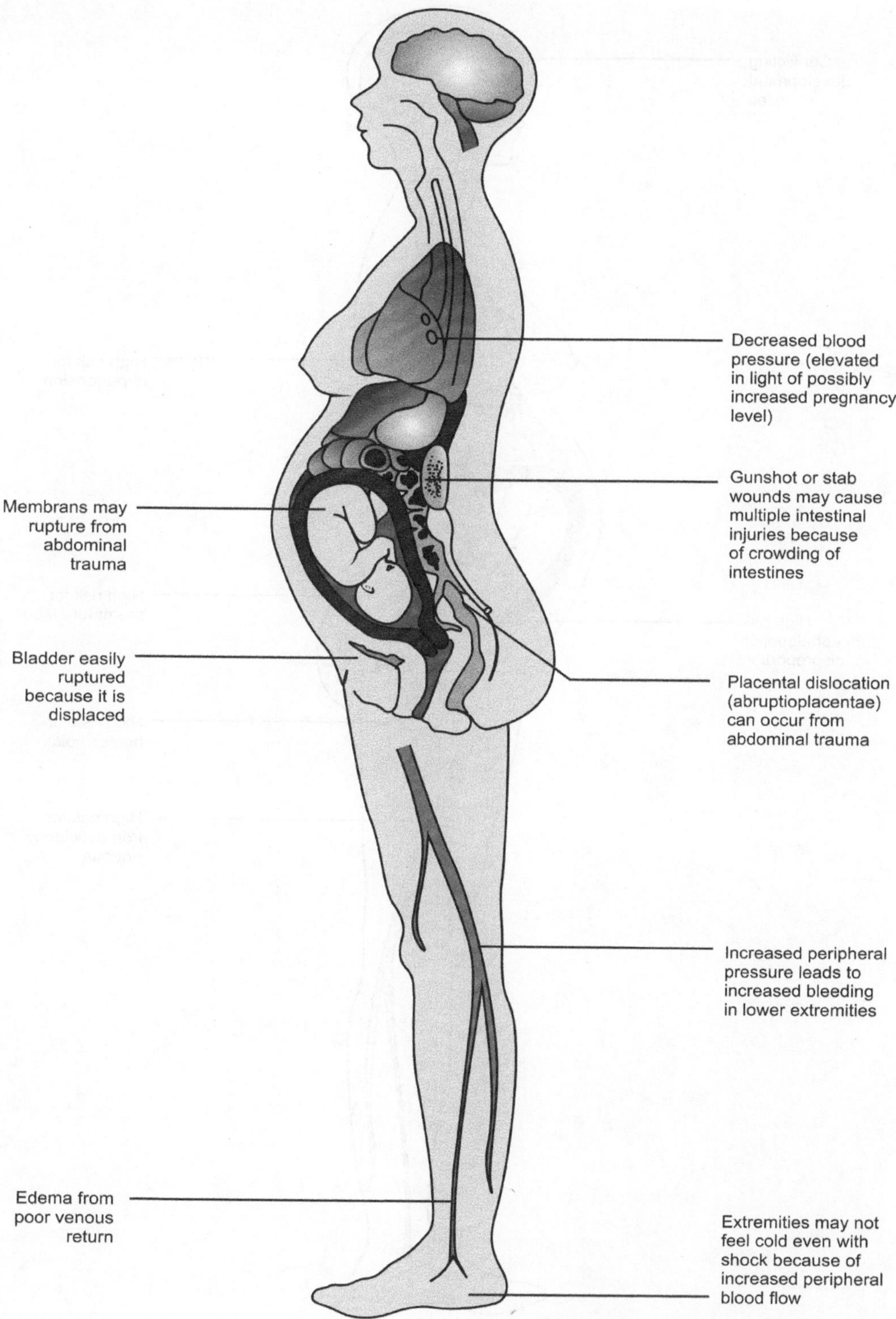

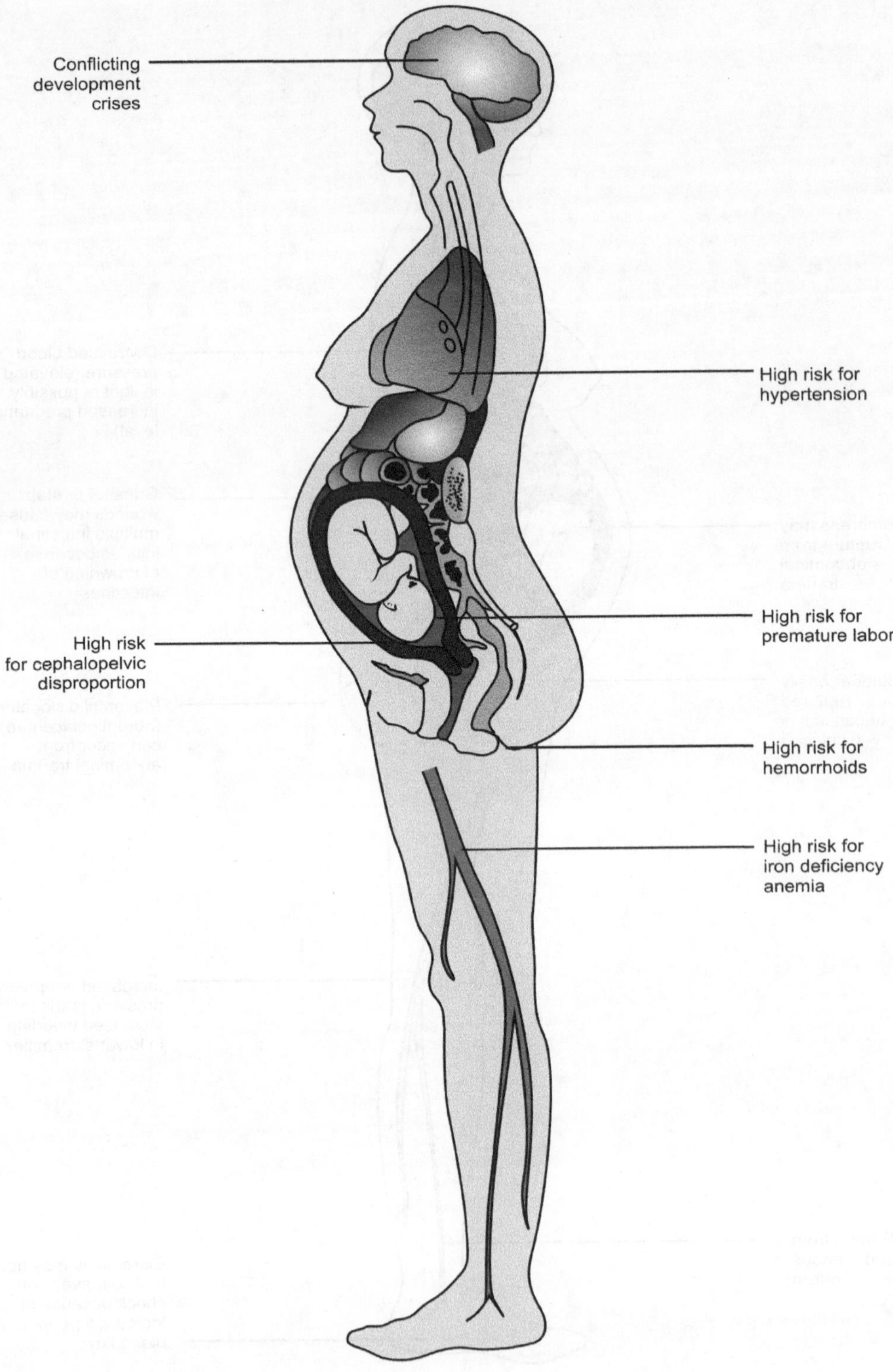
Conflicting development crises
High risk for hypertension
High risk for premature labor
High risk for cephalopelvic disproportion
High risk for hemorrhoids
High risk for iron deficiency anemia

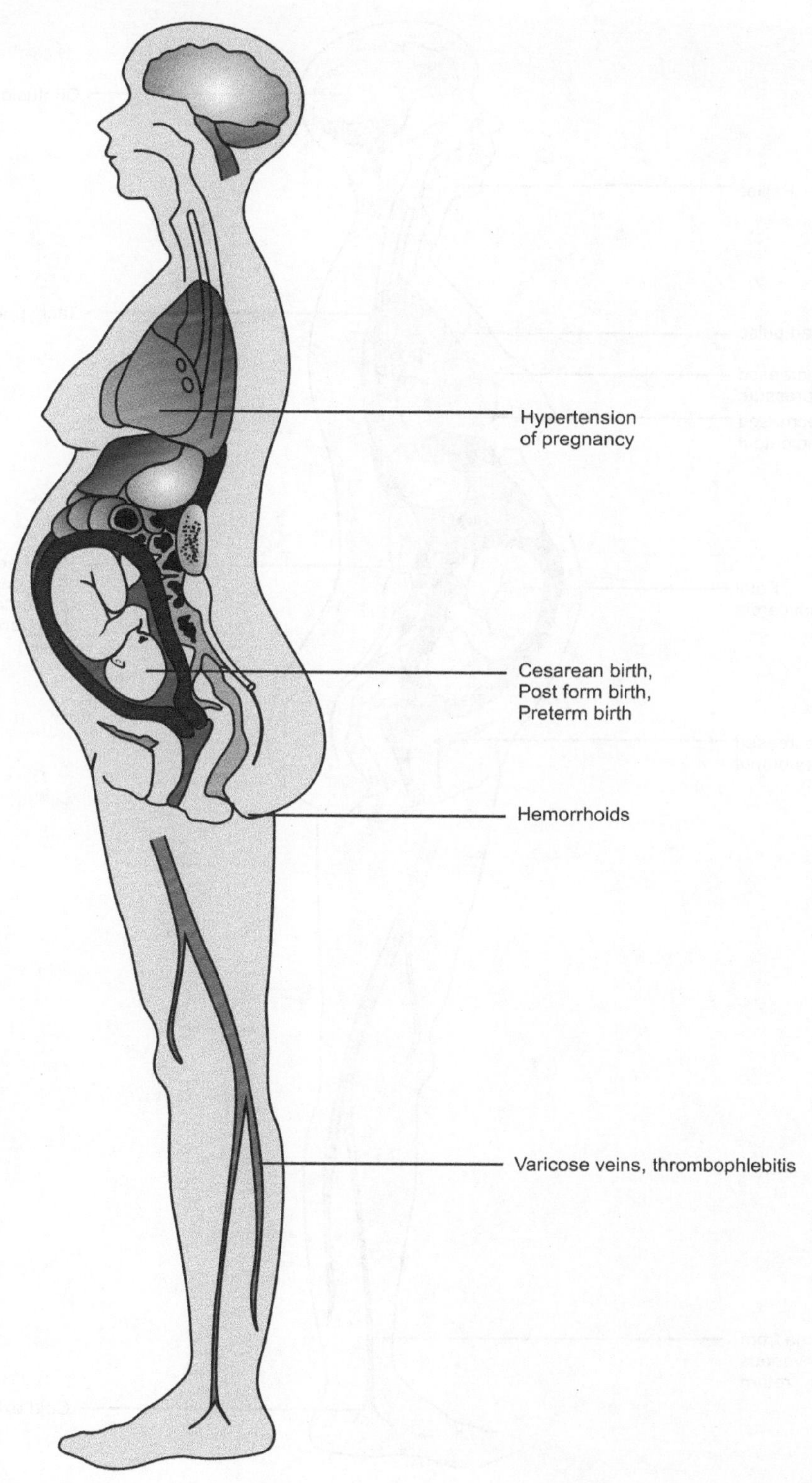
Hypertension
of pregnancy
Cesarean birth,
Post form birth,
Preterm birth
Hemorrhoids
Varicose veins, thrombophlebitis

ASSESSING THE PREGNANT WOMAN WITH HYPOVOLEMIC SHOCK

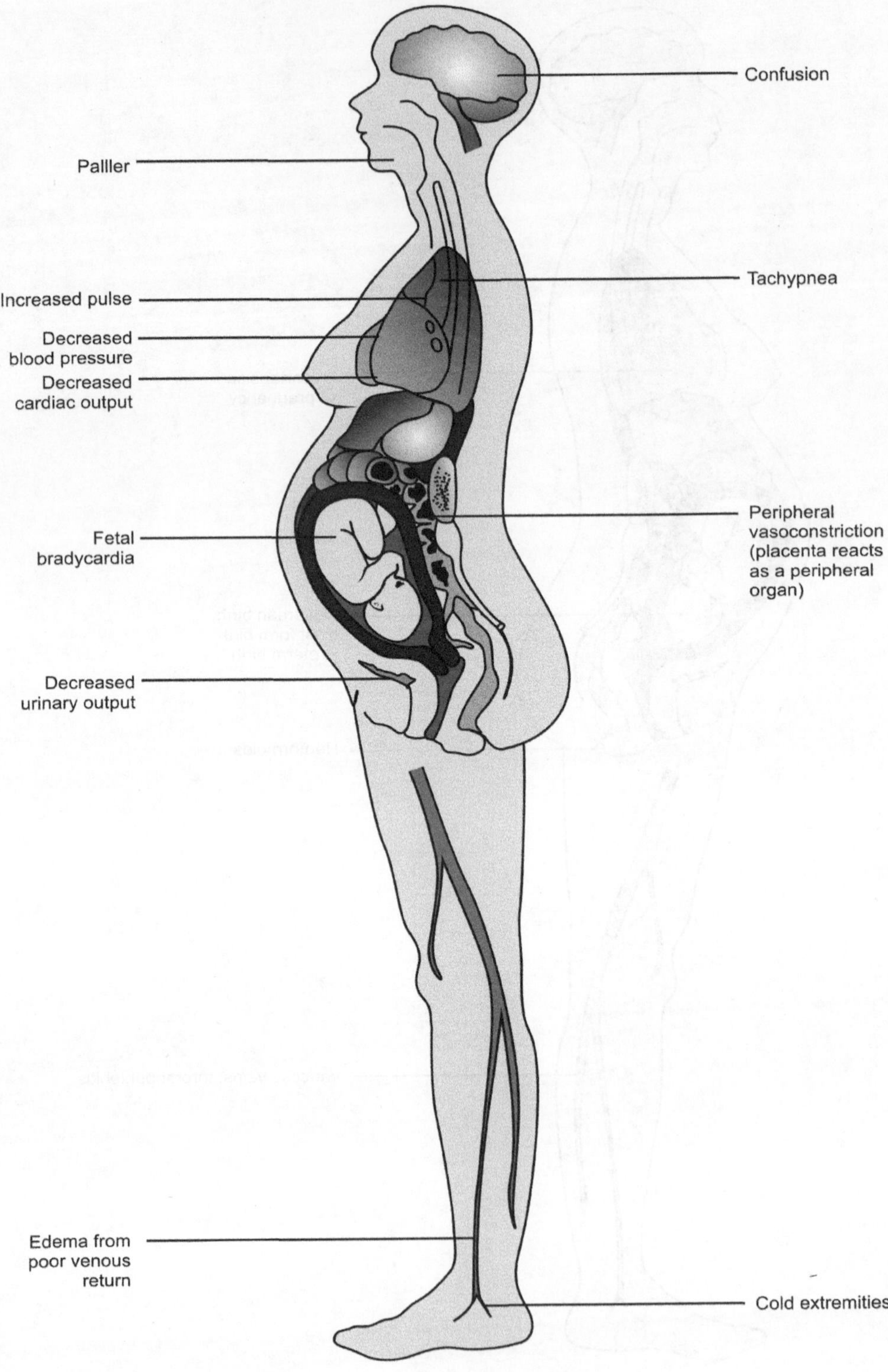

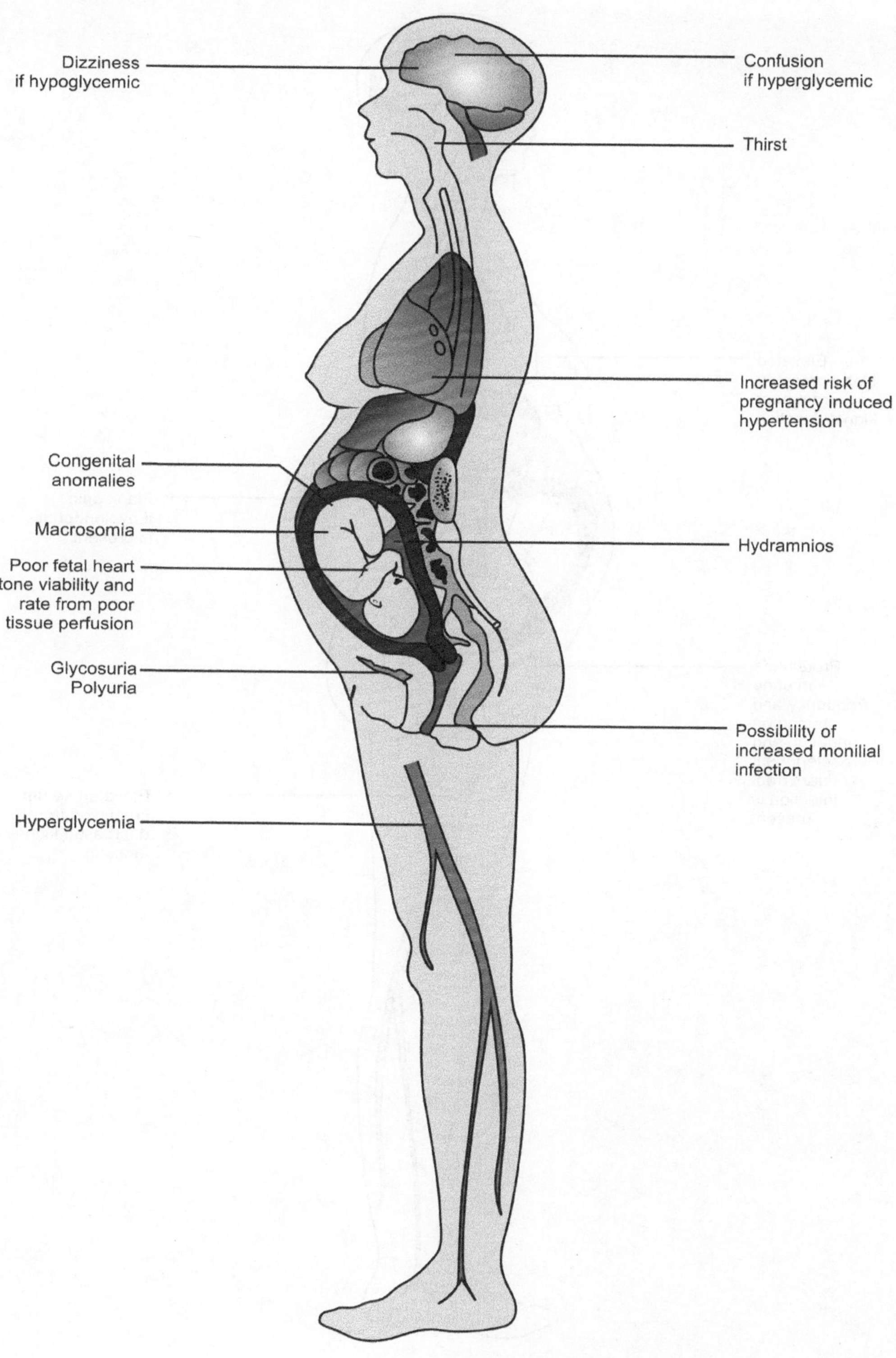
Dizziness
if hypoglycemic
Confusion
if hyperglycemic
Thirst
Increased risk of
pregnancy induced
hypertension
Congenital
anomalies
Macrosomia
Hydramnios
Poor fetal heart
tone viability and
rate from poor
tissue perfusion
Glycosuria
Polyuria
Possibility of
increased monilial
infection
Hyperglycemia

ASSESSMENT OF PREGNANT WOMAN WITH RENAL DISEASE

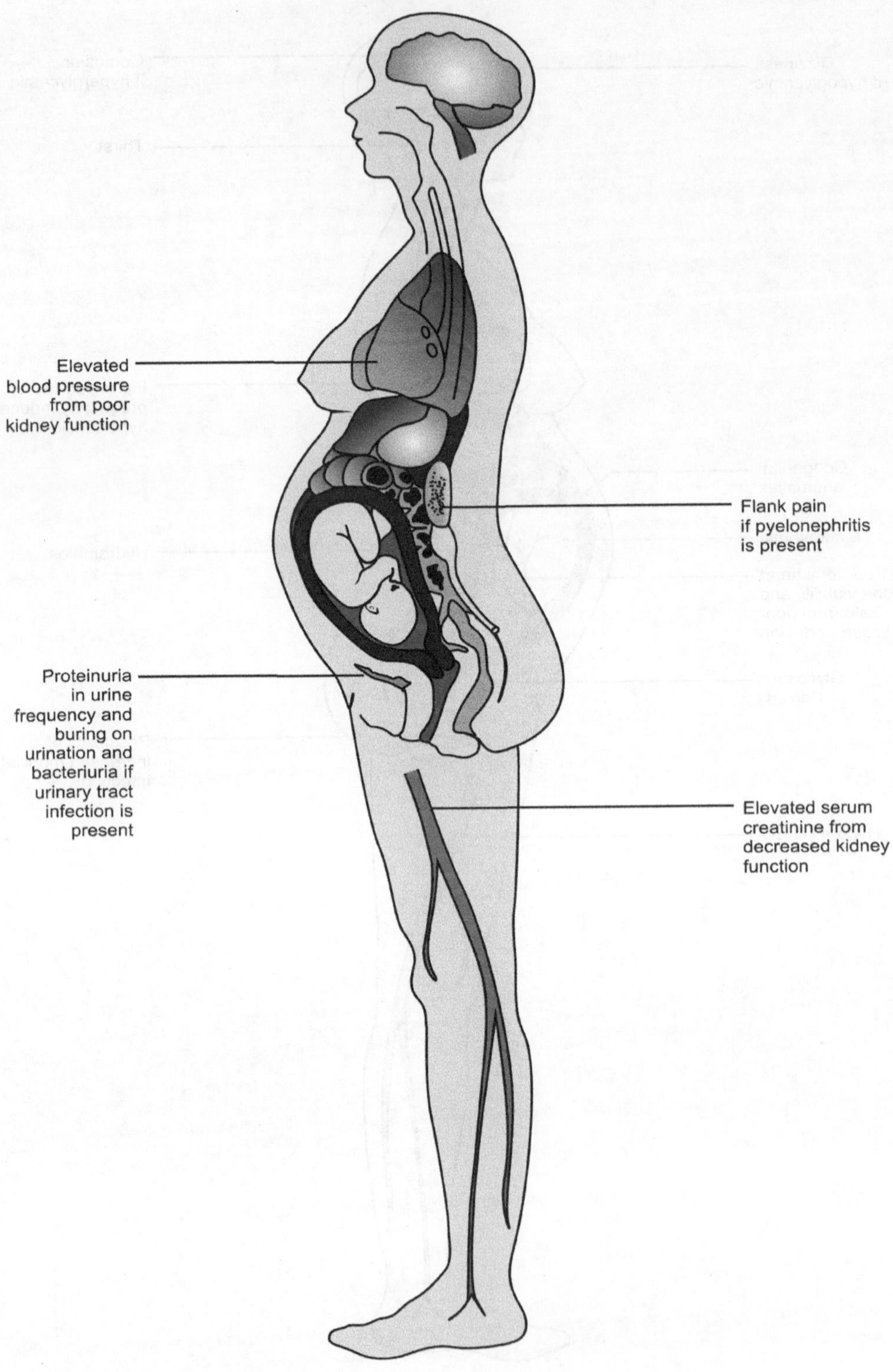

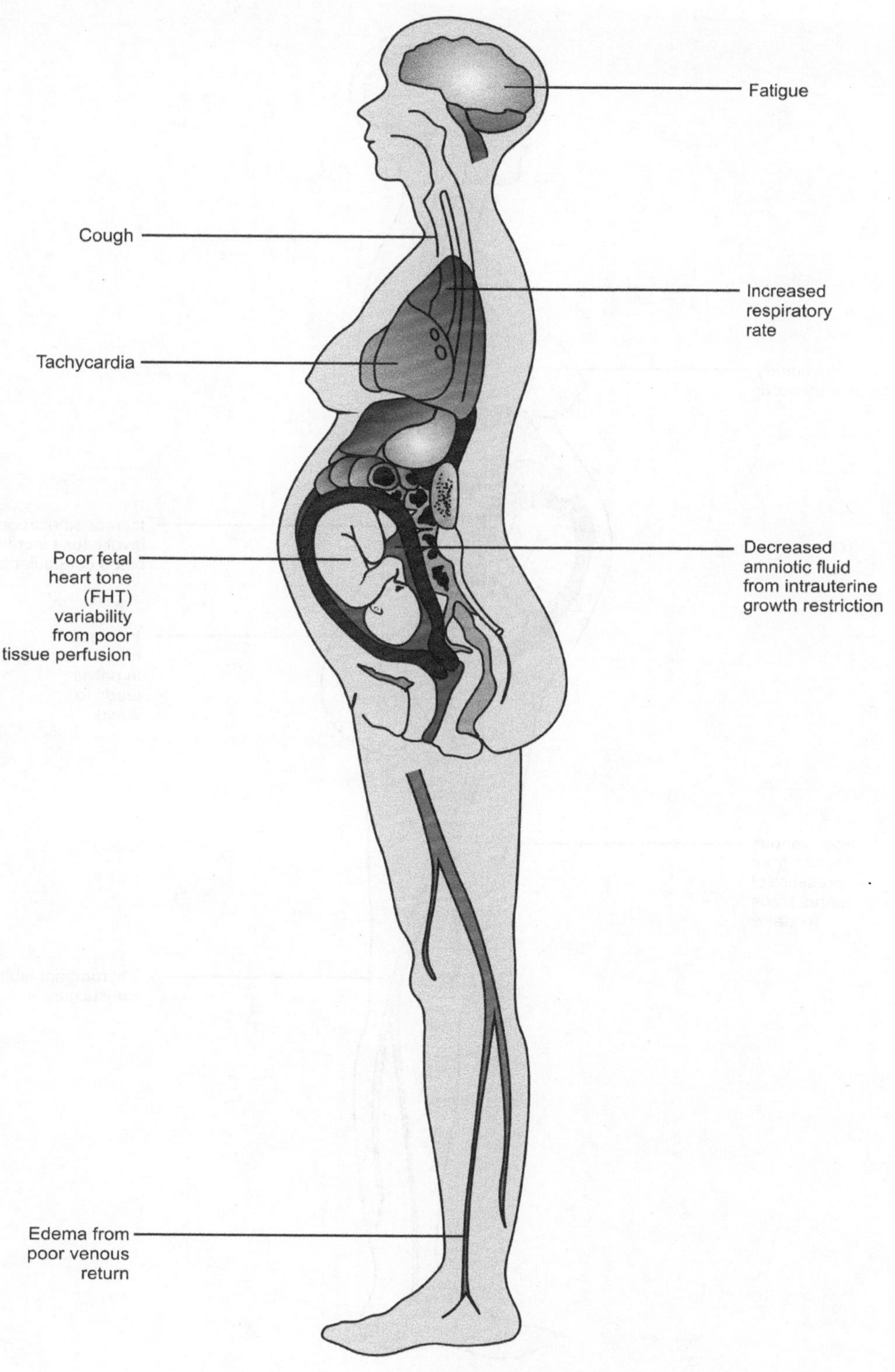
Fatigue
Cough
Increased respiratory rate
Tachycardia
Poor fetal heart tone (FHT) variability from poor tissue perfusion
Decreased amniotic fluid from intrauterine growth restriction
Edema from poor venous return

ASSESSMENT OF PREGNANT WOMAN WITH THROMBOEMBOLIC DISEASE

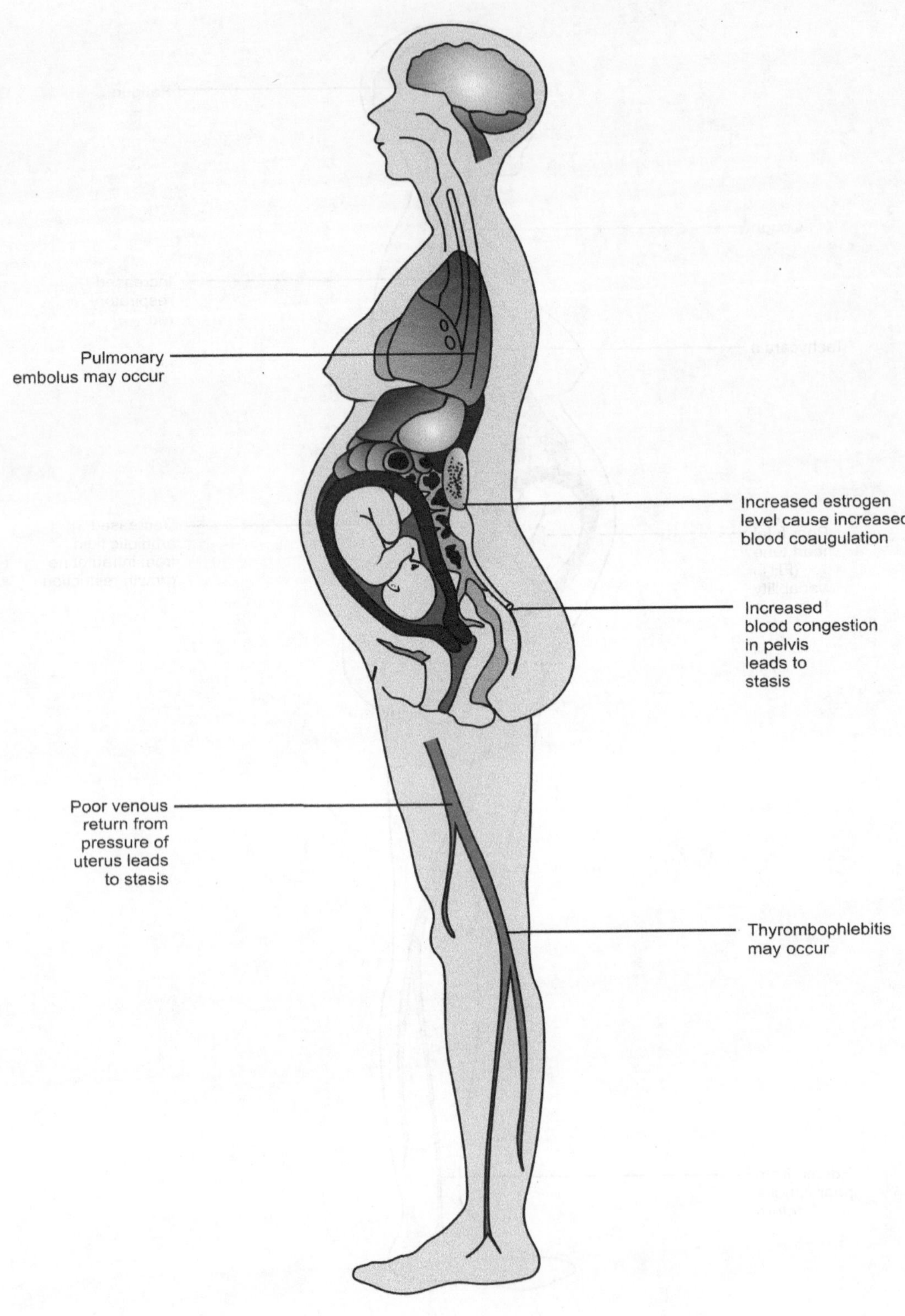

COMMON GYNECOLOGIC DISORDERS

Disorder	Possible Symptoms	Significance and Suggested Therapy
Vulva		
1. Cysts of skene or Bartholin glands	Asymptamatic swelling at the sides of the urinary meatus or vestibule	Such cysts are surgically incised to prevent blockage of gland duct.
2. Condylomata acuminata	Cauliflower like lesion on vulva	This lesion tends to occur in women with chronic vaginitis caused by epidermatrophic virus that causes common warts. Removed by cryocautery or knife excision.
3. Lichen sclerosus	Whitish papules on the vulva; asymptomatic	There is no need for removal; the area is biopsed because leukoplakia, a potentially cancerous condition, has an almost identical apperance.
4. Leukoplkia	Thick, gray, patchy epithelium that cracks; possibly a premalignant state that infects easily, accompanied by itching and pain	There by involves hydrocortisone and frequent return visits to health care personal [every 6 months] for observation to detect any changes suggestive of carcinoma
5.Carcinoma of the vulva	A shallow vulvar ulcer that does not heal	Vulvar cancer occurs most often in postmenopausal women represents only 3% to 4% of all reproductive tract cancers in women. Therapy is vulvectomy—vagina is left intact,and sexual relations and pregnancy,with cesarian birth to prevent tearing of fibrotic vulvar tissue,may be possible.
Vagina and Cervix		
1. Adenosis	Asymptamatic vaginal cysts with columnar rather than squamous epithelium present on vaginal walls.	This condition is caused by diethylstilbestrol [DES] administration, while in utero. has the potential for becoming malignant clear cell adeno carcinoma. If adenosis is present, an examination two or three times a year with a pap test and lugol's staining is necessary, and a woman should not use estrogen sources such as oral contraceptives. If adenocarcinoma occurs, local destruction of atypical cells can be achieved by excision,cautery,or cryosurgery. This condition is rarely seen today because DES is no longer prescribed during pregnancy.
2. cervical polyp	Red,vascular,protruding pedunculated tissue that bleeds readily with trauma	A polyp may be discovered because of vaginal spotting on coitus, tampon insertion,or vaginal examination. Removed vaginally by excision.Often associated with chronic cervical inflammation.
3. Cervicitis [erosion]	Reddened cervical tissue with whitish exudate	Documenting with a vinegar solution aids healing. May be treated with cryosurgery if extensive
4. Nabothian cyst	Clear shining circles on cervix from blacked gland ducts	No therapy is necessary.
5. Cervical carcinoma	Post coital spotting,unexplained vaginal discharge or spotting between menstrual periods	Cervical cancer is the most frequent type of reproductive tract malignancy; risk factors include coitus with multiple partners or uncirumcised males, herpes simplex 2 infections, or DES use during pregnancy.Diagnosed by pap test or colposcopy. Therapy is conization radiation or surgical excision.Pregnancy is possible following cervical carcinoma;cesarean birth may be necessary because of fibrotic cervical tissue, can be prevented by HPV vaccine.

Ovaries		
1. Endometrial cyst	Chocolate brown cyst on tender enlarged ovary; may cause acute pain if rupture occurs	Endometriasis is the cause;occurs in women aged 20-40 years. Therapy is surgical excision;ovary may or may not be removed depending on extent of cyst.
2. Follicular cyst	Amenorrhea and possibly dyspareunia;ovary tender and enlarged	Cysts typically regress after 1 or 2 months;low dose oral contraceptive may be prescribed for 6 to 12 weeks to suppress ovarian activity; estrogen may be continued for 6 months.
3. Poly cystic ovary syndrome	A syndrome of chronic follicular cysts	Excess testosterone by ovaries leads to inhibition of FSH and anovulation. Weight loss, reduction in triglycerides and cholestrol,and clomiphene citrate therapy to induce ovulation are used as therapy.
4. Corpus luteum cyst	Delayed menstrual flow followed by prolonged bleeding; ovary enlarged and tender	A corpus luteum persists rather than atrophies. Most regress in about in 2 months; a low dose of oral contraceptive may be prescribed for 6 weeks to suppress ovarian activity.
5. Dermoid cyst	Asymptamatic	Surgical resection
6. Carcinoma	Asymptamatic	Hysterectomy and salpingo oophorectomy.
Uterus		
1. Endometrial polyp leiomyomas	Intermenstrual bleeding	Removed by dilatation and curettage.
2. Endo metrial carcinoma	Vaginal bleeding between menstrual periods	Hysterectomy
3. Uterine prolapse	Vaginal pressure and low back pain	Surgery to repair uterine support or placement of pessary, a plastic uterine support.

BIOCHEMICAL TEST

It involves biologic examination and chemical determination procedures used to obtain the specimen for study include amniocentesis,PUBS,CVS and maternal sampling.

Test	Possible Findings	Clinical Significance
Maternal Blood		
Coomb's test	Titer of 1:8 and raising	Significant Rh incompatibility
Alpha-fetoprotein [AFP]	High levels after 15 weeks of gestation	Open neural tube defect
Amniotic Fluid Analysis		
Color	Meconium	Possible hypoxia or asphyxia
Lung Profile		
L/S ratio	>2:1	Fetal lung abnormality
Phosphatidyglyceral	Present	Fetal lung abnormality
Creatinine	>2 mg/dl	Gestation age > 36 weeks
Bilirubin	<0.015	Gestational age > 36 weeks, normal pregnancy, fetal hemolytic disorders
Genitic Disorders		
Sex linked Chromosomal Metabolic	Dependent on cultured cells for karyotype and enzymatic activity	Counseling possible require.

AMNIOCENTESIS

It is performed to obtain amniotic fluid which contains fetal cells.

PROCEDURE

Under direct USG visualization a needle is inserted trans-abdominally in to the uterus. Amniotic fluid is withdrawn in to the syringe. It is possible after 14 weeks of pregnancy when the uterus becomes an abdominal organ and sufficient amniotic fluid is available for testing.

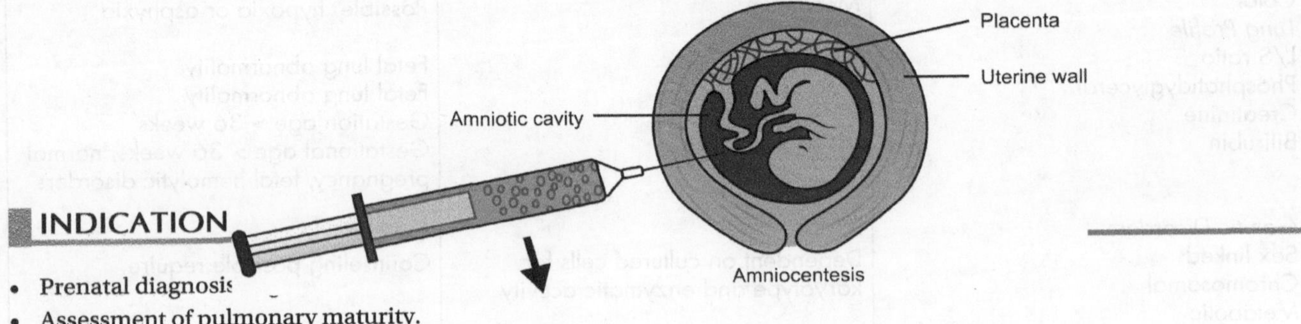

Amniocentesis

INDICATION

- Prenatal diagnosis
- Assessment of pulmonary maturity.
- Diagnosis of fetal hemolytic disease.

COMPLICATION

Less than 1 % of complication can occur.

In the Mother

Hemorrhage, infection, labor, abruptioplacenta, fluid embolism.

In the Fetus

Death, hemorrhage, infection, miscarriage, preterm labor, leakage of amniotic fluid.

CORDOCENTESIS

It is otherwise known as percutaneous umbilical blood sampling [PUBS]. Direct access to the fetal circulation during the second and third trimester.

PROCEDURE

Insertion of needle directly in to the fetal umbilical vessel under ultrasound guidance. Ideally the umbilical cord is punctured 1 to 2 cm from its insertion in to the placenta. At this point the cord is well anchored and will not move and the risk of maternal blood contamination is slight. Generally 1 to 4 ml of blood is removed and tested.

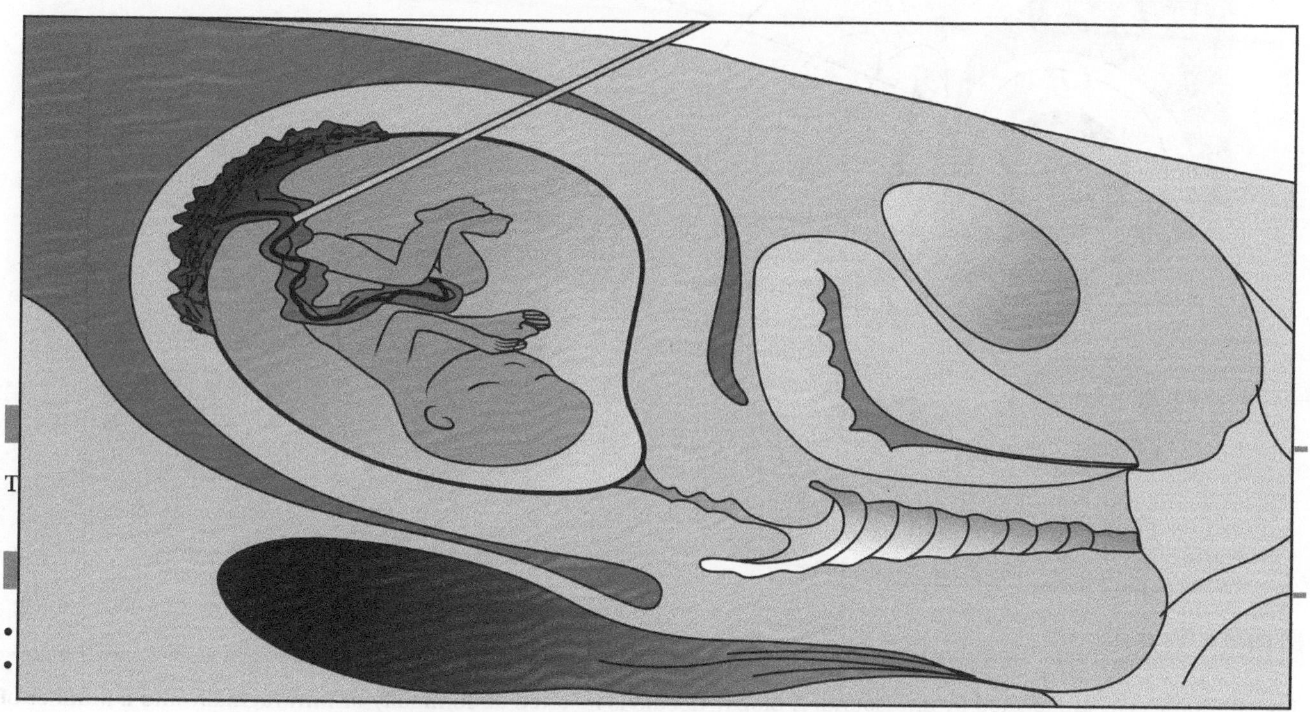

CHORIONIC VILLI SAMPLING

It is a diagnostic technique that involves the retrieval and analysis of chorionic villi from the growing placenta for chromosome or DNA analysis. It can be done as early as 5 week of pregnancy and commonly done at 8 to 10 weeks.

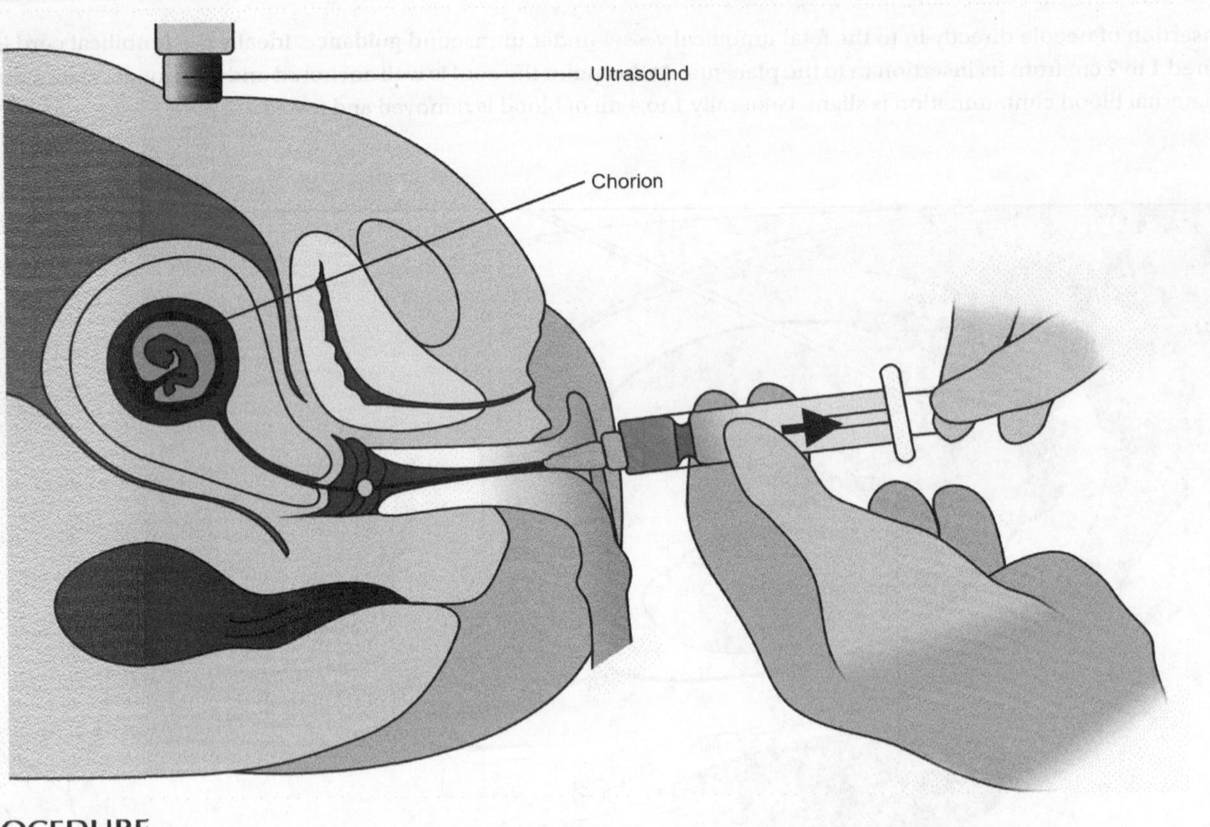

PROCEDURE

The chorionic cells are located by ultrasound. A biopsy needle is inserted abdominally or intravaginally and a number of chorionic cells are removed for analysis. Removed ones are karyotyped or submitted for DNA analysis.

INSTRUCTIONS

Instruct women to report chills or fever, threatened miscarriage.
Women with an Rh-negative blood type need Rh-immunoglobulin administration.

CRYOSURGERY

DEFINITION

This is a procedure where by destruction of the tissue is effective by freezing.

PRINCIPLE

It consists of a 'probe' the tip of which is cooled to a temperature below freezing point [-60 degree C].

Freezing produces cellular dehydration by crystallization of intracellular water ultimately death of cells. This is effective by rapid expansion of gas which is passed through it. Carbon dioxide is widely used while nitrous oxide and liquid nitrogen are also used.

INDICATION

1. Benign cervical lesions- such as CIN [cervical intraepithelial neoplasma], condyloma accuminata, leucoplakia, etc.
2. Condyloma accuminata of vulva and VIN [vulval intraepithelial neoplasma] diagnosed colposcopically and not more than 2 in size.
3. VAIN [Vaginal intraepithelial neoplasma], condyloma accuminata or vault granulation tissue following hysterectomy.
4. As a palliative measure to arrest bleeding in carcinoma cervix or large fungating recurrent vulval carcinoma.

TECHNIQUE

This is a outpatient procedure and is done without anesthesia.Commonly used technique is freeze-thaw-freeze.

Selection of probe is it should cover adequately the lesion. The probe tip is covered with water soluble jelly to provide good thermal contact with the cervix. First the probe is applied to the cervix and the freezing activated. When a good ice-ball extending 4 to 5 mm beyond the edge of the probe is obtained, the freezing is stopped: the probe thawed [to raise the temperature above freezing point] and removed. The probe which adhered to the tissue should not be pulled out until the temperature rises again. Usually 1 ½ to 3 minutes are required to obtain a satisfactory freeze. If necessary, a second time freezing technique may be employed to get a good result.

The application to the cervix freezes the tissue to a depth of about 3 mm.

ADVANTAGES

- Anesthesia is not required.
- Precise destruction of tissue.
- There is no secondary hemorrhage.
- Cervical stenosis is rare.

DISADVANTAGES

- Excessive discharge for about 2 to 3 weeks
- Healing is complete in 6 to 10 weeks.

KICK CHART

Kick chart is otherwise known as fetal movement chart. This chart will help us to find out of fetal activity by the mother, is simple yet valuable method for monitoring the condition of the fetus.

INDICATION

The fetus in pregnancy complicated by conditions that may affect fetal oxygenation.

METHOD

Ask the mother to count all fetal movements in a 12 hour period each day until a minimum of movements are counted.

Ask the mother to inform the health care people if the baby has not moved for 12 hours

The mother should take the kick chart along with her during the hospital visit.

Notes to remember by the nurse:

1. During the fetal sleep cycle the fetal movement will not present.
2. The fetal movement may temporarily reduce if the mother taken any depressant medication, smoking, alcohol.
3. The fetal movement does not decrease as the woman nears term.

KICK CHART

Days of the Week	Monday	Tuesday	Wednesday	Thursday	Friday	Saturday	Sunday
Date							
Kicks							
Date							
Kicks							
Date							
Kicks							
Date							
Kicks							
Date							
Kicks							

STANDARD LABORATORY VALUES IN PREGNANCY

Values	Pregnant	Normal
HEMATOLOGIC		
Hemoglobin	11.4-14 g/dl	12-16 g/dl
Hematocrit, Pcv,	32-42 %	37-47 %
Red Cell Volume	1900 ml	1600 ml
Plasma Volume	3700 ml	2400 ml
RBC	3.75-5.0 million/mm^3	4-5.5 million/mm^3
WBC	5000-15000 total per mm^3	4500-10000 total per mm^3
ESR	30-90 mm/h	0-20 mm/h
BLOOD COAGULATION AND FIBRINOLYTIC ACTIVITY		
Factors VII,VIII,IX,X	Increase in pregnancy,return to normal in early puerperium,factor VIII increases during and immediately after delivery	
Factors XI,XIII		
Prothrombin Time	Decrease in pregnancy	
Bleeding Time		60-70 sec
Coagulation Time	Slight decrease	1-3 min
Fibrinolytic Activity	No change	6-10 min
	No change	
Fibrinogen	Decreases in pregnancy, then abrupt return to normal	250 mg/dl
	400 mg/dl	
MINERAL AND VITAMIN CONCENTRATIONS		
Serum Iron	65-120 µg	75-150 µg
Serum Protein [Total]	5.5-7.5 g/dl	6.7-8.3 g/dl
Albumin	3.0-5.0 g/dl	3.5-5.5 g/dl
Globulin	3.0-4.00 g/dl	2.3-3.50 g/dl
Blood Sugar Fasting	65 mg/dl	70-80 mg/dl
2 Hour Post Prandial	Under 140 after a100 g carbohydrate meal is consider normal	60-110 mg/dl
CVS		
BP	114/65 mm of hg	120/80 mm of hg
Pulse Rate	80/min	70/min
Cardiac Output	6 l/min	4.5 l/min

CHEST RADIOGRAPH STUDIES		
Transverse diameter of Heart	1-2 cm increase	
Left border of heart	Straightened	
Cardiac volume	70 ml increase	
ECG		
V_1 AND V_2	Inverted T wave	
KV_4	Low T	
III	Q + Inverted T	
AVr	Small Q	
HEPATIC		
Serum Cholesterol	↑60 % from 16-32 weeks of pregnancy; remains at this level until after delivery	110-300 mg/dl
Serum alkaline phosphatase	↑from week 12 of pregnancy to 6 weeks after delivery	2-4.5 units
RENAL		
Bladder Capacity	1500 ml	1300 ml
Renal Plasma Flow	↑by 25%, to 612-875 ml/min	490-700 ml/min
GFR	↑by 50%, to 160-198 ml/min	105-132 ml/min
BUN	Decreases	25-40 mg/dl
Serum Creatinine	Decreases	20-22 mg/kg/24 hr
Serum Uric Acid	Decreases	257-750 mg/kg/24 hr
Urine Glucose	Present in 20% of gravidas	Negative
IVP	Slight to moderate hydroureter and hydronephrosis, right kidney larger than left kidney	Normal
MISCELLANEOUS		
Aldosterone	↑1mg/24 hr by third trimester	
Total Thyroxine Concentration	↑9-16 μg/dl thyroxine	5-1216 μg/dl thyroxine
Dehydroisoandrosterone	↑Plasma clearance tenfold to twenty fold	Plasma clearance 6-8 l/24 hr

NURSING DIAGNOSIS IN OBSTETRICS AND GYNECOLOGY

ANTENATAL

1. Altered nutrition pattern related to nausea and vomiting.
2. Urinary frequency and dysuria related to physiologic changes.
3. Anxiety related to pregnancy and a becoming a parent.
4. Health seeking behavior related to guidelines of pregnancy.
5. Risk for fetal injury related to knowledge deficit concerning possible fetal exposure to teratogens.
6. Imbalanced nutrition less than body requirement related to desire to control weight.
7. Decisional conflict related to choice of birth setting and birth process.

DURING LABOR

1. Pain related to uterine contractions and pressure on pelvic structures during labor.
2. Altered urinary elimination related to perineal edema and decreased bladder tone from fetal head pressure during labor and birth.
3. Ineffective coping pattern related to labor and delivery.
4. Anxiety related to hospitalization and birth process.
5. Knowledge deficit related to birth process.
6. Risk for injury related to prolonged labor with ineffective contractions and requiring oxytocin.

POSTNATAL

1. Pain related to physiologic changes in postnatal period.
2. Fluid volume deficit related to postpartum hemorrhage.
3. Risk for ineffective breast feeding related to anxiety and in experience.
4. Knowledge deficit related to postpartum care.
5. Pain related to development of mastitis.

CESAREAN SECTION

POSTPARTAL PERIOD

1. Pain related to surgical incision.
2. Risk for deficient fluid volume related to blood loss during surgery.

EXTENDED POSTPARTAL PERIOD

1. Constipation related to effects of abdominal surgery and anesthesia.
2. Impaired skin integrity related to surgical incision.
3. Fatigue related to effects of surgery.
4. Risk for fluid volume deficit due to postpartal fluid restriction.
5. Risk for impaired urinary elimination related to surgical procedure.
6. Risk for ineffective peripheral tissue perfusion related to immobility during and after surgery.
7. Risk for impaired parenting related to the emergent nature of birth or discomfort from surgery.

ADOLESCENT PREGNANCY

1. Altered family process related to the stress of adolescent pregnancy.

GENETIC RELATED

1. Health seeking behavior related to knowledge of possible genetic disorders of inheritance.
2. Situational low self esteem related to seeming inability to conceive.
3. Risk for altered fetal growth related to inadequate nutrition.

CONTRACEPTION

1. Health seeking behavior related to knowledge deficit concerning contraception.

NEW BORN

1. Impaired gas exchange related to immature pulmonary functioning.
2. Risk for deficient fluid volume related to insensible water loss at birth and small stomach capacity.
3. Risk for imbalanced nutrition, less than body requirements related to additional nutrients needed for maintenance of rapid growth, possible sucking difficulty and small stomach.
4. Risk for infection related to immature defense in preterm infant.
5. Risk for injury related to preterm labor and tocolytic therapy.
6. Risk for ineffective parenting related to infant's smaller than expected size, continuing rapid respirations, and birth marks.

THEORIES IN MIDWIFERY PRACTICE

INTRODUCTION

Quality care for all people continues to be nursing top priority. In forth coming centuries this goal is even more urgent than it has been because of the changing needs of the public, the conflicting priorities in health care professionals are confronting.

Practice based on theories allows for hypothesis about practice, which make it possible to derive a rationale for nursing actions. Practice based on science will suggest the image of nursing as a professional discipline.

DEFINITION

"Theory is a statement that purports to account for or characterize some phenomenon"

Barnum[1990]

"Theory is a systematic abstraction of reality that serves some purpose"

"Theory is a creative and rigorous structuring idea that project a tentative, purposeful and systematic view of phenomena"

-Chinn and Kramer [1991]

APPROACHES

Theories can be developed and tested through deductive, inductive or reproductive forms of reasoning. These approaches have been explicitly presented in the literature as systematic procedures for devising theory.

THEORIES IN MATERNITY

1. Reva Rubin Maternal Role Attainment Theory

Reva Rubin is a nurse midwife and her theory development has had a wide influence on the care of child bearing women.

Reva Rubin identified three aspects on maternity role:

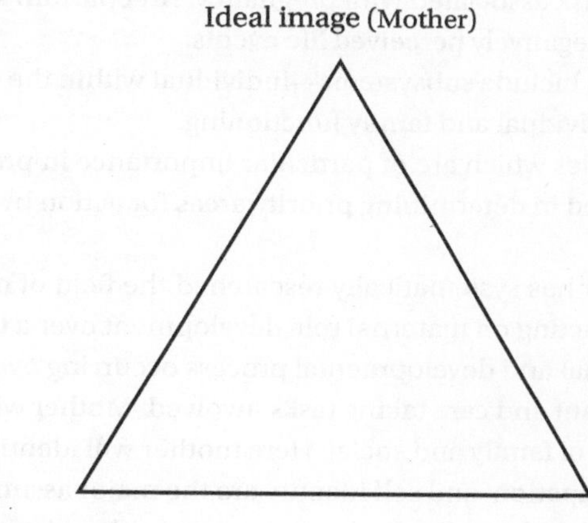

Special Notes

In 1967 Rubin described five operations or means by which maternal identity is incorporated in to the woman's image of herself. They are:

Talking on activities:

A. Mimicry: It is a replication of action and behaviors carried out by role models, e.g. other woman who are pregnant learning how pregnancy and delivery of baby.

B. Role play: Woman act out roles that they will be under taking in the future.

Talking in activities:

A. Fantasy: The woman imagines the future for herself, e.g. what the baby will wear and how the relationships with other members of the family.

B. Introjection and projection rejection: It is an active process in which the woman compares the available models with her view of herself and makes active decision about adopting or rejecting particular models, e.g. mimicry may occur when the mother is in a hospital she follows the technique which taught to her but introjections-projection and rejection will occurred when she is at home she follows her own approach [baby bath].

Letting go activities:

A. Grief work: It is a review in memory of the attachments and associated events of a former self. The experiences, interpersonal and situational associated with the former self include the actual and the hoped for the pleasant and unpleasant.

Concepts used in her theory:

Person: The woman and the development of the woman and her identity as a woman, mother and member of society who is mother—the central concern of the model is with the achievement by the woman of a positive identity as a mother.
Health: One of the tasks of pregnancy identified is the maintenance of safety of the woman and baby including maintenance of health.
Environment: In this maternal behavior as an activity which is demonstrated in interactions and relationships with others in the social system.
Nursing: The role of the midwife in this is to provide interventions which support the operations and achievement of the maternal tasks.
Rubin dealt the role attainment from the point of acceptance of the pregnancy to 1 month postpartum.

2. Ramona T Mercer'S Maternal Role Attainment Theory

Ramona T mercer is the only theorist whose work has been exclusively concerned with understanding the process of child bearing who is included in a collection considering the work of major theorists in nursing. Reva Rubin was her Mentor and she looked the role attainment beyond the period to 12 months postpartum.

Mercer has undertaken theory building and research in two main areas, they are:

- The effects of antepartum stress
- Attainment of the maternal role.
- **The effects of antepartum stress on the family:** Antepartum stress is described as resulting from a combination of negative life events and the level of risk associated with pregnancy. Antepartum stress is defined as a complication of pregnancy or at risk condition and negatively perceived life events.

The family is defined as systems which include subsystems—individual within the overall family system. These models consider antenatal stress in relation to individual and family functioning.

By testing this model regarding variables which are of particular importance in predicting the experience of antenatal stress on family functioning may be utilized in determining priority areas for action by midwives.

Attainment of the maternal role: Mercer has systematically researched the field of maternal role attainment and developed a complex model about factors impacting on maternal role development over a time.

In maternal role there is an interactional and developmental process occurring over a period of time, during which the mother becomes attachment with her infant and care taking tasks involved. Mother will develop confidence, competence, in the maternal role by supportive system of family and social. Here mother will identify herself as in maternal role.

Core self, mothering role, active participation, and self identity are the major assumptions in her research.

Model used in her theory: Mercer's model of maternal role attainment is placed within Bronfenbrenner's [1979] nested circles of the macro system, exosystem, and microsystem.

Macrosystem is generally explained about cultural consistencies.

Exosystem is including day care, parents work setting and school.

Microsystem is close to maternal role attainment. It includes mate relationship [father-mother relationship], family functioning, social support and stress.

Concepts used in her theory:

Person: Mercer refers a person here as a self or core self. It has the concepts of empathy, self concept, maturity, flexibility, attitudes, and pregnancy role attainments.

Health: It is a mother's and father's perception of their health, current health' health outlook, resistance –susceptibility to illness, health worry concern, sickness orientation, and rejection of the sick role. The health status of the family is negatively affected by ante partum stress.

Environment: Mercer does not define environment. She does however, address the individual's culture, mate, and family and or support network as it relates to maternal role attainment.

Nursing: According to mercer obstetrical nursing is the diagnosis and treatment of women's and men's responses to actual or potential health problems during pregnancy, child birth, and the postpartum period.

3. Ela Joy Lehrman: Components of Midwifery Practice

Lehrman is an American nurse midwife. By inductive and deductive theorizing she developed her concepts of the components of nurse midwifery practice. Three antenatal visits were audiotaped and from these she developed initial categories or concepts of practice. This is an approach to developing theory termed grounded theory which was developed by Glaser and Strauss.

Eight concepts of midwifery practice are:

- Continuity of care.
- Family-centered care.
- Education and counseling as part of care.
- Non-interventionist care.
- Flexibility in care.
- Participative care.
- Consumer advocacy.
- Time.

Lehrman provide a model which clearly indicates areas of midwifery activity. In the models developed by Mercer and Rubin midwifery practice has to be deduced. For example it can be deduced that to support the woman in mimicry activities relating to nutrition, the midwife has to provide information on diet in pregnancy, and support the woman in undertaking the activity. Lehrman provide a model of process or practice, while Mercer and Rubin provide a model of goals.

The maternal role development is achieved more easily within a system of midwifery care which provides family centered care, flexibility in care, lateral relationship and the other components of practice. Testing of relationships between these concepts will indicate the strength of the relationships that have been suggested

4. Ernestine Wiedenbach and the Need for Help

Ernestine wiedenbach developed a concept of nursing that was congruent with the prevailing ideas in late 1950s and early 1960s and that shifted nursing focus from the medical model to a patient model.

The theories addresses the central questions of, how do nurses help patients meet their needs? Help to wiedenbach is an integral part of nursing, and it is all actions that enable the individuals to overcome whatever hampers their ability to function. Help came in different ways ,one of which is in the form of intentional caring as differ initiated from help without caring.

Wiedenbach terms of realities of nursing:

The agent—the midwife: Raleigh [1989] and Wiedenbach's [1964] identified four elements in clinical nursing. They are philosophy, purpose, practice, and art. She comments that it cannot be assumed that all practioners hold the same philosophy, but this model is helpful in identifying the need to consider the beliefs of the individual midwife and the beliefs of colleagues.

The goal/purpose: According to wiedenbach the goal is to meet a person's need for help. A need for help is "any measure or action required and desired by the individual and which has potential for restoring or extending his ability to cope with the demands implicit in his situation".

Whenever a need for help exists, its presence may usually be suspected by behavior—physical, emotional, or physiological which is different from the usual pattern .The nurse midwife who is perceptive will be aware of it. Perceptiveness thus is an important attribute of postpartum nursing. The fact that a need is perceived, however, does not mean that it is met. First it must be identified, to do this requires skilled use of eyes, ears, hand, and mind. Eyes through which to observe or look intently; ears with which to listen expectantly; hands with which to feel; touch or palpate sensitively; and a mind with which to understand and interpret the observation. Once the need is recognized and has been validated by the one whose need it is, appropriate action may be taken to meet it.

The recipient: The recipient of care may be the childbearing woman, the family or the community who, for some reason or another are unable to meet their present needs. Nickel et al, comment that Wiedenbach's philosophy emphasis her respect for the individual.

The individual is seen as competent and able to determine if a need for help is being experienced. Nurses need to intervene only when there is an obstacle preventing the individual from satisfactorily coping with the demands placed up on her by the situation.

The means: The means of achieving the goal of midwifery care are expressed in practice of midwifery care are expressed in practice which comprises four phases;

i. Identification of the patient's experience need for help.
ii. Ministration of help that is needed.
iii. Validation that the help provided was indeed the help needed.
iv. Coordination of the resources for help provided.

The model identifies the need for the midwife to have knowledge, judgement and skills to enable the above steps of care to be achieved.

5. Jean Ball's Dech Chair's Theory of Emotional Well Being

Jean is a British midwife identified theory related to postnatal care such as role theory, change theory, theories of stress, cause and support system. This theory identified, that the maternal psychology depends on emotional well being of mother. It has three elements, such as:

i. Mother's personality[previous experience life crisis]
ii. Family peer support
iii. Maternal well being.

Factors affecting emotional well being:

- Perception of family support: postnatal ward atmosphere.
- Life events.
- Mother's self confident.
- Positive feeling after birth.
- Changing of life style/routine, satisfaction of motherhood.
- Mother's self image.
- Lack of sleep.
- Conflict activities.
- Partner support.
- Anxiety and support.

Theories under pinning midwifery practice:

- Parent child interaction—Barnard's theory.
- Cultural diversity—Leininger's theory.
- Preventive measures—Neuman's system model.
- Health promotion, belief 7 Behavior Model.
- Midwife and mother partnership peplau's theory.
- Psychological, physiological adaptation during pregnancy and postnatal Roy's adaptation theory.

NURSING RESEARCH AND BIOSTATISTICS

NURSING RESEARCH

UNIT I
Introduction

- Methods of acquiring knowledge –problem solving and scientific method.
- Research-definition, characteristics, purposes, kinds of research.
- Historical evolution of nursing research.
- Terms in research.
- Scope of nursing research.
- Health and social research.
- Concepts of evidenced based practice.
- Ethics in research.
- Overview of research process.

UNIT II
Review of Literature

- Importance, purposes, sources, criteria for selection of resources and steps in reviewing literature.

UNIT III
Research Approaches and Designs

- Types of research–qualitative and quantitative.
- Characteristics types advantages and disadvantages.
- Qualitative: phenomenology, grounded theory, ethnography.

UNIT IV
Research Problem

- Identification of research problem.
- Formulation of problem statement and research objectives.
- Assumptions and delimitations
- Identifications of variables.
- Hypothesis-definition, formulation and types.

UNIT V
Developing Theoretical/Conceptual Frame Work

- Theories ; nature, characteristics, purposes and uses.
- Using, testing and developing conceptual frame work, models and theories.

UNIT VI
Sampling

- Population and sample.
- Factors influencing sampling.
- Sampling techniques.
- Sample size.
- Probability and sampling error.
- Problems of sampling.
- Characteristics of a good sampling design.

UNIT VII

Tools and Methods of Data Collection

- Concepts of data collection.
- Data sources.
- Tools.
- Item analysis.
- Validity and reliability of tools.
- Pilot study.
- Procedures of data collection.

UNIT VIII

Implementing Research Plan

- Research plan design.
- Planning for data collection.
- Administration of tool.
- Interventions and collections of data.

UNIT IX

Analysis and Interpretation of Data

- Plan for data analysis.
- Preparing data for computer analysis and presentation.
- Statistical analysis.
- Interpretation of data.
- Conclusion and generalization.
- Summary and discussion.

UNIT X

Reporting and Utilizing Research Findings

- Communication of report-oral, written.
- Writing research report purposes, methods and style vancouver.
- Utilization of research findings.

UNIT XI

Critical Analysis of Research Reports and Articles

UNIT XII

Developing and Presenting A Research Proposal

BIOSTATISTICS

UNIT I

Introduction

- Definition.
- Types of data and its measurement.
- Uses of data.
- Organization and presentation of data.
- Tabulation of data.
- Frequency distribution.
- Graphical and tabular presentations.

UNIT II

Measure of Central Tendency

- Mean, median, mode.

UNIT III

Measures of Variability

- Range.percentiles.
- Average deviation.
- Quartile deviation.
- Standard deviation.

UNIT IV

Normal Distribution

- Probability.
- Characteristics and appilication of normal probability curve.
- Sampling error.

UNIT V

Measures of Relation

- Correlation.
- Regression.

UNIT VI

Significance of Statistics

UNIT VII

Use of Statistics in Psychology and Education

UNIT VIII

Health Statistics

UNIT IX

Uses of Computers in Research

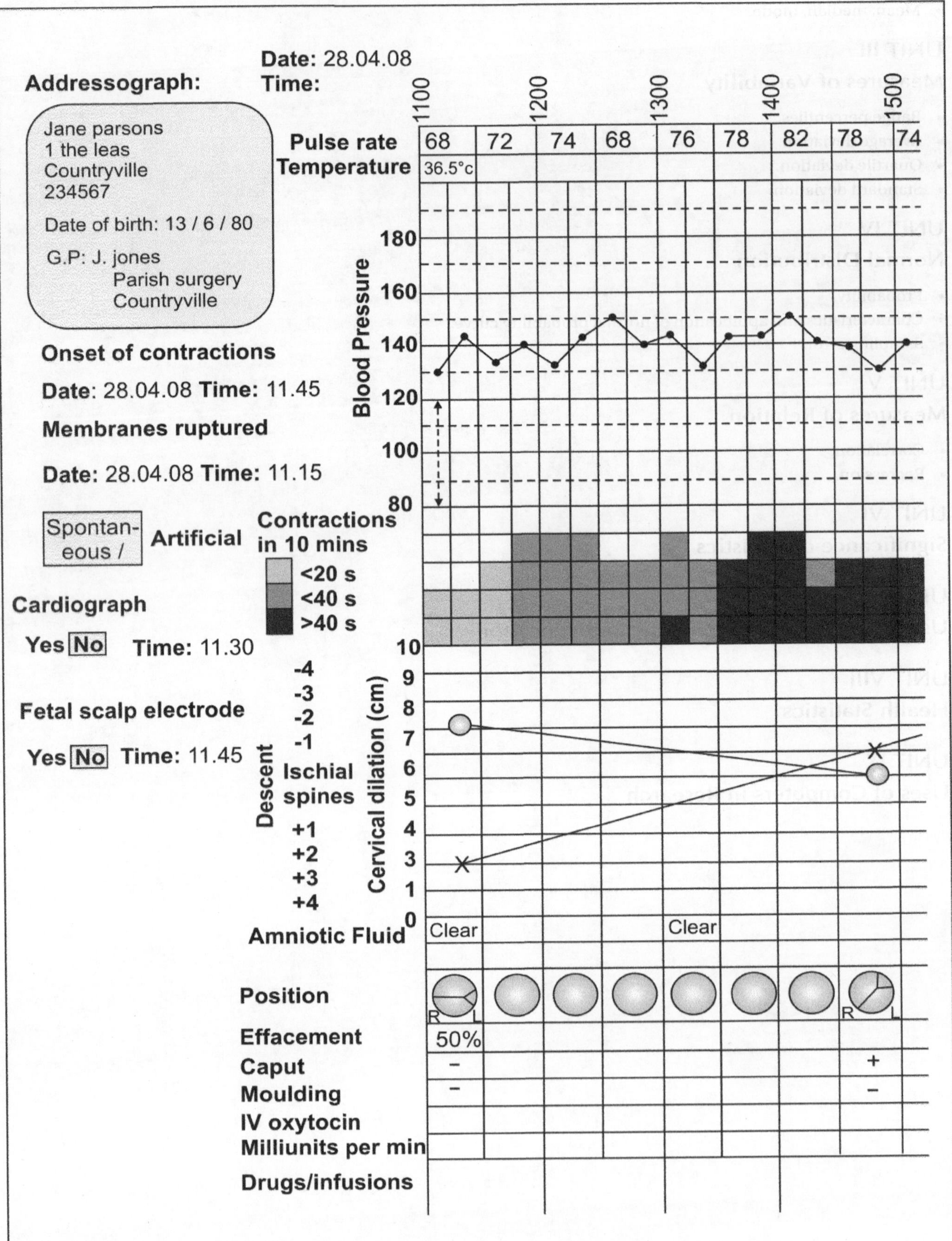

Example of partogram